Economic Impact of HIV/AIDS on Households

Economic Impact of HIV/AIDS on Households

Savio P. Falleiro

www.sagepublications.com
Los Angeles • London • New Delhi • Singapore • Washington DC

First published in 2014 by

 SAGE Publications India Pvt Ltd
B1/I-1 Mohan Cooperative Industrial Area
Mathura Road, New Delhi 110 044, India
www.sagepub.in

SAGE Publications Inc
2455 Teller Road
Thousand Oaks, California 91320, USA

SAGE Publications Ltd
1 Oliver's Yard, 55 City Road
London EC1Y 1SP, United Kingdom

SAGE Publications Asia-Pacific Pte Ltd
3 Church Street
#10-04 Samsung Hub
Singapore 049483

Published by Vivek Mehra for SAGE Publications India Pvt Ltd, typeset in 10/13 pt Palatino by Diligent Typesetter, Delhi, and printed at Saurabh Printers Pvt Ltd, New Delhi.

Library of Congress Cataloging-in-Publication Data

Falleiro, Savio P.
 Economic impact of HIV/AIDS on households / Savio P. Falleiro.
  pages cm
 Includes bibliographical references and index.
 1. AIDS (Disease)—Economic aspects. 2. HIV infections—Economic aspects. 3. AIDS (Disease) in children—Patients—Family relationships. 4. HIV-positive persons—Family relationships—Economic conditions. I. Title.
  RA643.8.F343   362.19697'92—dc23   2014   2014005758

ISBN: 978-81-321-1359-1 (HB)

The SAGE Team: Shambhu Sahu, Archa Bhatnagar, Anju Saxena and Rajinder Kaur

To Sameena, Samara and my parents;
and to all those infected and affected by HIV/AIDS

Thank you for choosing a SAGE product! If you have any comment, observation or feedback, I would like to personally hear from you. Please write to me at <u>contactceo@sagepub.in</u>

—Vivek Mehra, Managing Director and CEO,
SAGE Publications India Pvt. Ltd, New Delhi

Bulk Sales

SAGE India offers special discounts for purchase of books in bulk. We also make available special imprints and excerpts from our books on demand.

For orders and enquiries, write to us at

Marketing Department
SAGE Publications India Pvt. Ltd
B1/I-1, Mohan Cooperative Industrial Area
Mathura Road, Post Bag 7
New Delhi 110044, India
E-mail us at <u>marketing@sagepub.in</u>

Get to know more about SAGE, be invited to SAGE events, get on our mailing list. Write today to <u>marketing@sagepub.in</u>

This book is also available as an e-book.

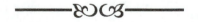

Contents

List of Tables   ix
List of Figures   xv
List of Abbreviations and Acronyms   xvii
Preface   xix
Acknowledgements   xxiii

1   About HIV/AIDS   1

2   Income and Employment   13

3   Inflow and Outflow of Household Income   59

4   Health and Medical Expenditure   119

5   The Way Ahead   169

Appendix I: Sample Profile   186
Appendix II: Income and Employment   197
Appendix III: About the Study   200
Glossary   206
References   211
Index   222
About the Author   230

List of Tables

2.1i	Households sample profile vis-à-vis annual HH income	15
2.2i	Employment status, income-slabs and number of years since death of dead AIDS HH members	20
2.2ii	Details pertaining to the dead AIDS members	21
2.3.1i	Past and present employment status of the HIV+ respondents	25
2.3.1ii	'Change in job' status of HIV+ respondent after HIV detection	25
2.3.1iii	Reasons for leaving job, whether received benefits and number of times changed jobs	26
2.3.1iv	Amount received by those who got financial compensation at the time of leaving the job	27
2.3.1v	Notable job changes: Past and present	28
2.3.1vi	Monthly income slabs of those employed at time of HIV detection and now	30
2.3.1vii	Monthly income of the earlier and present employment of the HIV+ respondents	31
2.3.1viii	Nature of change in earnings from the time of HIV detection to present earnings	31
2.3.2i	Employment, discrimination and employer-support of presently employed HIV+ respondents	33
2.3.2ii	Whether earning HH members lost income last year due to sickness-caused absenteeism	35
2.3.2iii	Days of sickness-contributed absenteeism of those currently working	35
2.3.2iv	Income lost due to illness-caused absence during the last one year	36

2.4i	Need for a caregiver in the HH	38
2.4ii	Months since caregiving required, age of CGs and amounts lost due to caregiving	38
2.4iii	Identity, employment, occupation and age of CGs, and whether lost income due to caregiving	39
2.4iv	Details of CGs currently not employed	41
2.4v	Amount lost per month by CGs who were working earlier	41
2.5i	Details of dead non-HIV earning members of the last two years	43
2.5ii	Distribution of dead non-HIV earning members based on monthly income slabs	44
2.6.1i	Coping mechanisms related to income and employment made use of in HIV/AIDS HHs	46
2.6.2i	Details of HIV+ members or CGs who lost job/income during the last one year	48
2.6.2ii	Income lost and months not working	49
2.6.2iii	Total income lost last year due to loss of job on account of HIV/AIDS	49
2.6.2iv	Total income lost last year vis-à-vis total annual HH income of concerned HHs	50
2.6.3i	Details of those losing two income sources	52
2.6.3ii	Summarized details of HIV/AIDS HHs pertaining to loss of income	53
3.1.1Aa	Comparative monthly food expenses	63
3.1.1Abi	Regular monthly HH consumption expenditure details of HHs actually incurring the expenses	69
3.1.1Abii	Comparative regular monthly HH consumption expenditure details of all sample HHs	70
3.1.1Abiii	Comparative regular monthly HH consumption expenditure slabs (excluding food)	76
3.1.1Aci	Comparative 'other annual HH consumption expenditure' details for concerned HHs	77
3.1.1Acii	Comparative 'other annual HH consumption expenditure' details of all sample HHs	80
3.1.1Aciii	Comparative distribution of HHs based on 'other annual HH consumption expenditure'	83

3.1.1B	Comparative amount of remittances in the last one year	85
3.1.1Ci	Comparative savings/investments (including modes of savings) in the last one year	87
3.1.1Cii	Comparative details of HHs which saved and dissaved at the same time	89
3.2.1A	Comparative distribution of sample HHs based on annual HH income slabs	93
3.2.1B	Distribution of HHs for total amount raised since HIV detection and annual HH income	95
3.2.1Ba	Comparative dissavings (including its forms) in the last one year	99
3.2.1Bb	Comparative borrowings in the last one year	102
3.2.1Bc	Comparative profile of UUI of the last one year	104
3.2.1Bc⁺i	Summarized details related to borrowings and UUI	105
3.2.1Bc⁺ii	HHs opting for borrowings, UUI or both during the year despite no dissavings	107
3.2.1Bc⁺iii	Amounts raised through dissavings and borrowings post HIV detection	108
3.2.2	Comparative total amounts raised through dissavings, borrowings and UUI in the last year	109
4.2i	Comparative profile of HHs vis-à-vis total 'other annual HH consumption expenditures': *With* and *without* total annual HH medical expenditures	123
4.2ii	Distribution of sample HHs in terms of 'other annual HH consumption expenditure': *With* and *without* total annual HH medical expenses	124
4.2iii	Distribution of sample HHs on the basis of total annual HH medical expense slabs	125
4.3i	Comparative profile of sample HHs vis-à-vis NHIE/NHIT	127
4.3ii	Comparative number of days sick last month excluding those frequently/continuously sick	128
4.3iii	Comparative profile of sample HHs vis-à-vis treatment to those sick in the last month	129

4.3iv	NHIT and number of years since detection of HIV	130
4.3v	NHIT of those frequently or continuously sick in the last month	132
4.3vi	Treatment of those frequently/continuously ill with NHIE and years since HIV detection	133
4.3vii	Comparative figures on duration of NHIT and days bedridden and not gone for work	133
4.3viii	Comparative figures of NHIT expenses of sample HHs of the last one month	134
4.3ix	Distribution of sample HHs in terms of total expenses on NHIT in the last one month	135
4.3x	Distribution of sample HIV/AIDS HHs based on total NHIT expense and annual HH income	137
4.4i	Hospitalization details of HIV+ respondents including number of times hospitalized	138
4.4ii	Comparative profile of sample HHs vis-à-vis HIE/HIT	139
4.4iii	Comparative figures of number of times and days hospitalized in the last one year	141
4.4iv	Comparative figures of hospitalization expenses of sample HHs of the last one year	142
4.4v	Comparative total HIT expense slabs of sample HHs in the last one year	143
4.4vi	Distribution of HIV/AIDS HHs sample based on total annual HIT expenses and HH income	144
4.5.1ai	Whether HIV+ respondents take ART	147
4.5.1aii	Details pertaining to ART-related monthly expenses	148
4.5.1b	Comparative RMMT expenditures *excluding* ART expenses	150
4.5.2i	Summarized figures of HIV+ respondents and their RMMT including ART	152
4.5.2ii	Comparative total RMMT expenditures of sample HHs	153
AI.i	Profile of HIV/AIDS sample HHs	186

AI.ii Comparative profile of sample HHs based on
profile of HH head and total annual HH income 187

AI.iii Comparative profile of sample HHs on
the basis of employment of HH heads 189

AI.iv Employment and educational qualifications of
HH members excluding the HH head 191

AI.v Descriptive statistics of sample HHs 192

AI.vi Comparative profile of sample HHs on
the basis of basic facilities used 193

AI.vii Comparative profile of sample HHs based
on ownership of items 194

AI.viii HIV status of HH head 195

AI.ix Profile of HIV+ respondents 195

AI.x Age description of sample HIV+ respondents 196

AII.i Age and employment of the dead AIDS
members 197

AII.ii Summarized details of present and past
employment status of CGs 199

AII.iii Coping mechanisms adopted and total annual
HH income slabs 199

List of Figures

1.1   Year-wise number of HIV+ cases
reported/detected in Goa   5

3.1.1Ab   Comparative distribution of regular monthly
HH consumption expenditure including food   74

3.1.2   Where and how the HH rupee goes during
the year   90

3.2.1Bc[+]   Distribution of HIV/AIDS HHs vis-à-vis
revenue raised post HIV detection   108

3.2.2   How and from where the HH rupee comes from   110

3.3.1   Modes of dependence of HIV/AIDS HHs for
covering expenses/deficits during the year   111

List of Abbreviations and Acronyms

AIDS	Acquired Immunodeficiency Syndrome
ART/ARV	Anti-retroviral Treatment [or therapy]/Anti-retroviral
BPL	Below Poverty Line
CG	Caregiver
Chap.	Chapter
CSW	Commercial Sex Worker
C&S Home	Care and Support Home
ET	*The Economic Times*
F	Females
GDP	Gross Domestic Product
GNP	Gross National Product
GSACS	Goa State AIDS Control Society
HAART	Highly Active Anti-retroviral Therapy
HH	Household
HIE/HIT	Hospitalized Illness Episodes/Treatment
HIV	Human Immunodeficiency Virus
HIV+	HIV-positive
HRLN	Human Rights Law Network
ICTC	Integrated Counselling and Testing Centre
ILO	International Labour Organization
M	Males
Max.	Maximum
MDG	Millennium Development Goals
Min.	Minimum
MTCT	Mother-to-Child Transmission
N	Number/Total/No.
NACO	National AIDS Control Organisation

NACP	National AIDS Control Programme
NCAER	National Council of Applied Economic Research
NFHS	National Family Health Survey
NGO	Non-Governmental Organization
NI	National Income
NHIE/T	Non-hospitalized Illness Episodes/Treatment
OI	Opportunistic Infection
p.a.	Per annum
PC	Personal Computer
PLHA	Person/People Living with HIV/AIDS
PLWH	People Living with HIV
PLWHA	People Living with HIV/AIDS
p.m.	Per month
Q-S	Questionnaire/Schedule
R&D	Research and Development
RMMT	Regular Monthly Medical Treatment
SD	Standard Deviation
Sec.	Section
STD/STI	Sexually Transmitted Diseases/Infections
TB	Tuberculosis
TOI	*The Times of India*
TV	Television
UNAIDS	Joint United Nations Programme on HIV/AIDS
UNDP	United Nations Development Programme
USAID	United States Agency for International Development
UUI	Unrequited and/or Unrevealed Income
WFPR	Work Force Participation Rate
WHO	World Health Organization

Preface

Ever since the detection of human immunodeficiency virus (HIV), millions of lives have been lost worldwide to acquired immunodeficiency syndrome (AIDS), with a large number surviving the disease living a life of extreme penury, despair, squalor and hopelessness. Often listed as a major health emergency, HIV/AIDS has had serious and overwhelming effects on human development, with the scale of the epidemic even contributing in some instances to the collapse of informal social safety nets. Besides taking lives, HIV/AIDS has separated families, reduced life expectancy (by as much as 10–20 years in some countries), destroyed and impoverished communities and, to a significant extent, undermined progress of the Millennium Development Goals (MDGs). In India, projections on mortality from infectious diseases predict that by the year 2033, HIV/AIDS could cause 22 per cent of all deaths and 40 per cent of deaths from infectious diseases (Nielsen and Melgaard 2004: 47). Literature unequivocally records HIV/AIDS widening the economic divide between households (HHs), making better-off HHs poor and poor HHs poorer; with the fallouts particularly being severe on poor/marginalized and female-headed HHs. Adverse impacts involving social, psychological, legal, political, ethical and economic dimensions, among others, affect people with HIV/AIDS. The economic fallout itself is broadly categorized into three groups: micro/individual/HH level, sectoral level and macro/national level. It is said that the impact of HIV/AIDS felt at the individual/HH level could significantly influence the impact at the other levels and to that extent the most immediate response in impact alleviation interventions need to start with the affected individuals and their households (Gupta and Panda 2002: 184).

This book addresses an issue of international, national and local importance; an issue where the predominant attention is the humanitarian and developmental catastrophe that it is often accused of leading to, particularly in the developing world. Acknowledging the dearth of empirical studies particularly on the HIV/AIDS front in Goa, and considering the serious nature of impacts that HIV/AIDS bear on individuals/HHs, government and society, it was felt that an attempt to systematically document the economic fallout of this debilitating illness was the need of the hour. The pursuit of this goal led to systematic and concerted efforts involving, among others, extensive field research, detailed interviews and personal in-home surveys. This book is an outcome of an in-depth analysis involving 400 HHs: 200 HIV/AIDS HHs and 200 non-HIV/AIDS HHs. Considering the nature of the study and its implications on the society at large, it was felt that besides publishing the findings in research journals (accessible primarily to researchers), there was a need to present them in an easy-to-read book so as to reach a wider audience.

In India, where the impact of HIV/AIDS is not much visible due to the low prevalence rate and huge population, it is important to study both the human and economic dimensions of the disease (Ojha and Pradhan 2006: v). While the present study/book, with its focus on the micro-level impacts on HHs and individuals in the economically productive and socially active age group of 18–60 years, is in line with the above-mentioned objective; it also conforms largely with two important arguments for having socio-economic impact studies: as a tool for *advocacy* and as a precursor for *planning*—a rationale for prevention and mitigation (see Barnett and Whiteside 2000: 11). The study/book, the first of its kind in Goa, besides being of great assistance to researchers in hypotheses formulation and in the conduct of longitudinal forms of studies on account of its elaborate and in-depth description of the ground situation through quantitative and qualitative information, can assist policy-makers as well, in broadly assessing the (in)adequacy of the existing measures provided by the government and others such as non-governmental organizations (NGOs) and foreign donors with reference to HIV/AIDS. This study/book would help towards making suitable changes to the existing initiatives in order to address deficiencies and improve the day-to-day living of 'people living with HIV/AIDS' (PLWHA) and their HHs. The study/book additionally shows whether HHs are able to cope with (and if so, how) the peculiar conditions they face of rising expenditures and falling incomes post HIV infection. By making a comparative analysis with a matched non-HIV/AIDS HHs sample, the study/book brings to light the finer complexities and the real-life situation of HIV/AIDS HHs and provides an objective insight into areas where HIV/AIDS HHs are at a greater disadvantage— areas which therefore need more urgent attention. The study/book also addresses issues where significant gender-based hardships exist; issues which call for a more focused corrective mechanism. Suggestions on future role that the government, NGOs, corporate bodies and others could play for effectively tackling HIV/AIDS and in alleviating the sufferings of the HIV/AIDS individuals/HHs is another positive outcome of this study. Notwithstanding the fact that this study/book is one of its kind in Goa, in high probability it is one of the rare studies anywhere as well to focus on the critical role played by 'partly/fully sponsored' food and 'unrequited and/ or unrevealed income' (UUI) in HIV/AIDS HHs. The uniqueness of the research methodology/design adopted towards analyzing HH income/expenditure and health/medical expenditure provides perspectives that may not yet be available in other studies.

In the context of Goa, this book will be highly useful since, with no other similar work being available, it can assist in framing effective/appropriate strategies considering the ground situation, which in many ways is different from other Indian states. It is important to be reminded that Goa (with a population of 1.3 million at the time of the study) is a *moderate prevalence* state as regards HIV/AIDS, bordered by *high prevalence* states; further, Goa has the potential for high risk on the HIV infection front on account of its socio-economic, geographic and cultural background. The tourism-dependent coastal state of Goa, with relatively Westernized and non-conservative lifestyle, has often been headlined as being a sex and drug haven. Until recently, as high as three HIV-positive (HIV+) cases were detected on an average in Goa daily, that too at the Integrated Counselling and Testing Centres (ICTCs) alone.

The book is presented in five chapters. While the first deals with broad introductory issues pertaining to HIV/AIDS, the last brings out concluding remarks and the 'the way ahead'. The three intervening chapters highlight the study findings, with one chapter each focusing on income/employment, inflow/outflow of HH income and health/medical expenditures. Keeping a wider audience in mind, unnecessary use of technical jargon and statistical values has been avoided; for example, wherever statistical significance was found at the 99, 95 or 90 per cent level, the same has been shown in easy-to-understand terms like *very/ highly significant, significant* and *quite significant,* respectively. Likewise, the absence of statistical significance at even the 90 per cent level has been indicated as *absence of significance.* Some broad 'ground' perspectives of the study/book which may be of interest to discerning research-oriented readers are provided under Appendices.

Savio P. Falleiro

Acknowledgements

This book has been an outcome of an intensive study, one made possible by the blessings and divine guidance of God almighty, besides the assistance, support and encouraging words of some wonderful people who fatefully came along as inspirational partners. Without this informal collaboration, this ambitious study, considering its numerous inherent constraints, would not have been a reality.

This book/study would not have seen the light of day if not for the direction of my mentor Dr (Mrs) Silvia M. de Mendonça e Noronha (Professor, Department of Economics, Goa University); my ever grateful thanks to her for the belief and motivation. My sincere thanks to all academicians (in)directly involved with my work, including the ever-obliging and modest, Dr P.K. Sudarsan and Dr Pranab Mukhopadhyay (Associate Professors, Department of Economics, Goa University).

Had it not been for the cooperative staff of numerous HIV/ AIDS-associated NGOs, my work would not have progressed as smoothly. My deep and profound gratitude to some extraordinary human beings who always went out of their way to assist me; my sincere gratitude in particular to Rev. Sr Vinita (FMCK) and Mrs Crecy Baptista for the invaluable inputs and timely assistance. Thanks also to Sr Francisca, Sofia, Joy, Maya and Mahesh; not to forget Roy Gomes, Ranjan and Roselle Solomon, Azad, Viency, Vishranti, Upa, Hari, Srinivas and Laxmi; besides Chetan and Felicio. My humble gratitude also goes to the doctors who assisted me with advice and contacts, especially the ever-willing and affable Dr Rajesh G. Naik. With deference to the wishes of a number of individuals, particularly those associated with NGOs, who did not want to be named (leave aside acknowledged), I humbly say a silent *Thank You* to each one.

The present study would not have been possible if not for the co-operation of HIV-positive persons (and often their family members as well); my heartfelt thanks to each respondent who without compulsion or *quid pro quo* spent precious time with me, without letting the dreaded stigma get into the way of a comprehensive and meaningful interaction. My gratitude also to those from non-HIV/AIDS households who willingly consented to participate in the study.

A sincere word of thanks to my former Principal, Rev. Dr Walter de Sá, during whose term this study was initiated, and to my present Principal, Rev. Dr Simão R. Diniz, for his constant support and encouragement. Thanks also to Diocesan Society of Education (DSE), University Grants Commission (UGC), library staff of various institutes, faculty members of various departments of Goa University, acquaintances (for the invaluable references and hyperlinks in particular) and to my own college colleagues and students for all the support.

My gratitude to the publishers of this book and to the editors/ publishers of research journals which published articles related to the study. A sincere note of acknowledgement to all the authors whose works have been cited in this book and listed under *References* section; their contributions have indeed been a source of enrichment with regard to the existing body of knowledge pertaining to the subject. A special word of acknowledgement to Pradhan et al. associated with the UNDP/NCAER/NACO report/ study of 2006.

Last but not the least, my heartfelt gratitude to Sameena and Samara; their constant and unflinching support helped make the entire journey (of the study) into an enjoyable experience. To those whom I have failed to acknowledge my gratitude, *mea culpa*; my apologies for the unintentional lapse—the responsibility of the same rests entirely on me (likewise any errors, omissions and editorial *faux pas* which may have inadvertently crept in while preparing this book). May God bless us all.

1

About HIV/AIDS

Just as a stone thrown into a pond will create ripples that reach to the farthest edges of the pond, so too will the effects of HIV infection be experienced at all social, cultural and economic levels (Reid 2000a: 19).

HIV/AIDS has been a scourge globally, particularly in the developing world. Figures of infected persons have increased from about 2 million in 1985 to a phenomenal high of around 40 million by just about the fifth year of the new millennium. According to more recent figures, the number of HIV/AIDS-infected people worldwide is pegged at around 33.3 million (UNAIDS 2010). It has been claimed that ever since the beginning of the epidemic over 20 million people have died of AIDS—the equivalent of a world war (D. Broun, in Human Rights Law Network [HRLN] 2008: 26).

The United Nations Development Programme (UNDP) *2005 Human Development Report* identified AIDS as the factor inflicting the single greatest reversal in human development history (UNAIDS 2006: 82). The Center for Disease Control defines AIDS as any HIV+ person having one or more of the 21 AIDS-defining *opportunistic infections* (OIs) (S. Mehra, in HRLN 2008: 34). The *cluster of differentiation 4* or commonly called CD-4 count test is also an indicator of whether an HIV+ individual has progressed to AIDS. In case of a normal person the CD-4 count is in the range of 700–1,500 per cubic millilitre of blood (Singhal and Rogers 2006: 47). When this count comes below 500 in case of HIV+ individuals, it is reflective of a depressed immune system; when it falls below 200 (or CD-4 percentage becomes less than 14 per cent), the person is said to be having AIDS, with he or she developing episodes of

OIs (ibid.; Bora 2008: 274; Singh 2003: 82). According to a World Bank report (2000), most patients succumb to OIs within two years after the onset of AIDS.

While HIV/AIDS was first detected in India in 1986, globally it was first detected in the USA in 1981. Since the syndrome was first detected among gays, it was initially called *gay-related immunodeficiency* (GRID) (Pavri 1996: 2). HIV was first discovered by Francoise Barre-Sinoussi, Luc Montagnier[1] and colleagues at the Institut Pasteur, Paris, in 1983; with contributions coming also from Popovic, Gallo and co-workers in 1984. The virus of AIDS, that is HIV, was originally called *lymphadenopathy associated virus* (LAV) and *human T lymphotropic virus-III* (HTLV-III) (ibid.: 29). Controversy with regard to the name was settled by the International Committee for Nomenclature of Viruses, with the virus (recognized as a *lentivirus*) being given the name of human immunodeficiency virus, that is, HIV (ibid.).

Claimed to be the single largest infectious killer (Kakar and Kakar 2001: 230), according to *2006 AIDS Epidemic Update*, a joint report of UNAIDS and WHO, somebody is infected somewhere or the other with HIV every eight seconds, with another 8,000 dying every day.[2] As high as 95 per cent of those who contract the virus each day are from developing countries (Bloom et al. 2001a: 8). Two-thirds of those infected with HIV live in Sub-Saharan Africa (Avert 2008), with the disease spreading in other regions, especially East Europe, Caribbean, and parts of East and South Asia. Children born in six African countries are not expected to reach the age of 40 years; in Sub-Saharan Africa, over a third of the adults could constitute the HIV population within 10 years (Drummond and Kelly 2006: 6). The AIDS epidemic in some countries is so severe and devastating that according to Red Cross and Red Crescent it needs to be classified as a disaster, that is, an event beyond the scope of any single society to cope with (Foulkes 2008). Incidentally, AIDS, which was first recognized in industrialized countries where most of the funding for research, prevention and care was concentrated, has expanded fastest in poor countries, where socio-economic and political mechanisms that keep countries poor act together to produce a situation in which AIDS thrives (WCC 2002: 97–98).

There are three chronological stages in the AIDS epidemic: AIDS-initiating, AIDS-impending and AIDS-impacted (Sharma 2006: 166). An HIV/AIDS epidemic is a long and slow process as the virus acts slowly with an incubation period of many years; by the time that even a few infected people are recognized with AIDS, many more live whose condition has not been diagnosed (Barnett and Whiteside 2000: 8). AIDS cases are only the most visible part of a much larger HIV-infected population; though debatable, it was estimated earlier that for each actual case there were likely to be an additional 50–100 infected individuals (Sinha 1995: 28).

HIV/AIDS, still spoken in hushed tones, is spreading across all sections of society. The seriousness of the problem made the Indian Army to contemplate making pre-recruitment HIV screening compulsory. Similarly, governments of Goa, Andhra Pradesh, Maharashtra and other Indian states deliberated upon to make HIV test mandatory before registration of marriage. Until as recent as less than a decade back India was claimed, by no less than agencies like UNAIDS and WHO, and accepted by the Indian government, to be the country with the dubious record of having the maximum number of 'people living with HIV/AIDS' (PLWHA) in the world. India had 5.7 million of the 8.6 million people living with HIV in Asia—most of them incidentally were aged between 15 and 49 years (Sinha 2006b: 1). These figures look grimmer if one realizes that one out of every 100 Indian adults or 0.9 per cent of the total adult population were HIV+;[3] or that the 0.9 per cent itself got translated into 0.4 million AIDS deaths in India in 2005 (Rashid 2006: 1) and that India is home to 60 per cent of South Asia's HIV patients (Sinha 2006a: 13).

Although the HIV *prevalence rate*[4] appears to be low in India, the actual figures in absolute terms are high due to India's massive population where even a small fraction of 0.1 per cent gets translated into a big number of infected persons. HIV/AIDS epidemic in India is characterized as a *concentrated epidemic*, concentrated mainly in certain states, and in these states within certain districts; it is not a *general epidemic* as in South Africa, Sub-Saharan Africa or Botswana where the prevalence rates are 18–32 per cent (K. Sujatha Rao, in HRLN 2008: 14).[5] It needs to be mentioned that in the context of India the true extent of the HIV/AIDS situation is difficult to assess, especially considering the mammoth size of a billion plus population, that majority of the deaths taking place each year occur outside a hospital setting where cause of death is often unrecorded, and with many dying without even knowing their HIV+ status.

Ever since about 2006–2007, as per the relatively more recent announcements of National AIDS Control Organization (NACO) and supported by UNAIDS and WHO, the figures of HIV+ cases have been reduced by almost half in India. This change was attributed to adoption of presumably more accurate modes of estimation unlike earlier methods. The figure of infected persons consequently came down from 5.7 million to a range of 2–3.1 million; and from a percentage figure of 0.9 to 0.36 per cent.[6] According to National Family and Health Survey (NFHS–3) the prevalence rate stood even lower at 0.28 per cent (Dhar 2007: 9). The reduction in figures changed India's dubious first rank of HIV infected population to third, next to South Africa and Nigeria (Ramachandran and Rajalakshmi 2009: 23; Sinha 2007: 6). Incidentally, the reduction in figures of PLWHA in India was not without dissenting voices. According to Jain and Stephens (2008: 17) the fall in numbers did not represent a decline in the number of PLWHA; it only represented a change in the way they were counted.

Based on the analysis of the Sentinel Surveillance data from year 2000, the states and union territories in India were initially classified into three groups: high, moderate and low HIV prevalence states, depending upon the prevalence rates among the high-risk population groups and antenatal women (Panda et al. 2002: 25; Ramamurthy 2004: 231–232; Shaukat and Panakadan 2004: 159–160). Incidentally, even within the low prevalence states there are areas where the problem is heightened (A. Kehra, in HRLN 2008: 29). Of late the mentioned classification has been increased to four groups with the 'low prevalence' group being divided into two: 'highly vulnerable states' (Group III) and 'vulnerable states' (Group IV) (GSACS 2008: 3; 2009: 6). Out of 610 districts in the country, 187 have been identified as high prevalence (A. Kehra, in HRLN 2008: 29).

HIV/AIDS was first detected in Goa in 1987. Ever since, there have been an increasing number of PLWHA in Goa (see Figure 1.1). While prior to 1992 there were very few HIV cases detected ranging from 3 to 30 per year, post-1992 has seen the number rising steadily with more than 800 cases being detected each year since the year 2000 (GSACS 2005–2006: 7), with there being an average of three cases detected per day since 2004 at the state-monitored Integrated Counselling and Testing Centres (ICTCs) alone. According to Goa State AIDS Control Society (GSACS 2010), as of November 2010, the total number of HIV cases detected in Goa since 1987 were 13,387; reported AIDS death cases up to October 2010 were 747; and number of people estimated with HIV was 16,000. There were as of November 2010, 1,370 AIDS cases reported in Goa (ibid.).

Majority of the HIV/AIDS cases in Goa are located in the coastal belt and in the four *taluka*s of Marmagoa, Salcete, Bardez and Tiswadi (GSACS 2009: 12 and 17). Incidentally, these talukas are relatively well developed, economically and socially, as compared to the other seven talukas of Goa. In Goa, while the disease is prevalent more in men, it is the females of younger age group that

Figure 1.1

*Year-wise number of HIV+ cases reported/detected in Goa^*

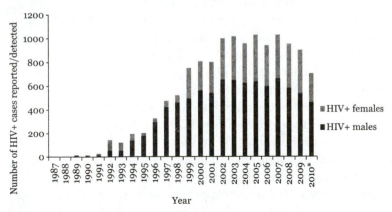

Year

Source: GSACS (2010).
Notes: ^Graph prepared as per the data provided by GSACS (2010).
*Figures are as of the month of November 2010 only.

are infected more (GSACS 2009, 2010). NACO considers Goa to be among the *moderate prevalence* states; bordered by *high prevalence* states of Maharashtra and Karnataka; with South Goa district being one of the high prevalence districts in India.[7] Sexual mode of HIV transmission accounts for as high as up to 96 per cent of the infected cases in Goa (*Economic Survey, 2005–2006*: 73; GSACS 2010).

Notwithstanding official statistics of HIV/AIDS infected persons in India/Goa, the actual numbers could be much higher since there would be many more whose HIV+ status has not yet been detected. Death certificates are inaccurate source of data for AIDS-related mortality because the cause of death in AIDS patients is rarely given as AIDS, but is often camouflaged as one of OIs (Schoub 1995: 212). Figures available for HIV infections are usually estimates; for definite statistics each and every one will have to be tested (D. Broun, in HRLN 2008: 25–26). Of the estimated PLWHA only 17 per cent know they are HIV+ (K. Sujatha Rao, in HRLN 2008: 16). Stigma and discrimination, besides those going to private doctors/clinics for check-ups and treatment, make it difficult to know who the infected persons are.

Most PLWHA are in the prime productive and reproductive age group of 15–44 years. About half of all HIV infections occur among young people below 24 years of age, indicating the inherent vulnerability of youth in most cultures, a fact which is constant even though there are many different contexts within each culture (WCC 2002: 15). In India, 89 per cent of the reported HIV cases have been in the age group of 18–40 years, with over 50 per cent of all new infections taking place among young adults below the age of 25 years (Verma and Roy 2002: 79). In Goa as of September 2009, 87 per cent of the HIV-detected cases were among those in the 15–49 years age group (GSACS 2009: 17).

Contrary to the earlier perception, it has now been realized and accepted that children and those in rural areas are among the more adversely affected groups. As Medhini et al. (2007a: 562) highlight, while HIV infects approximately 1,800 children under the age of 15 each day, 15 million children under the age of 18 had already lost at least one parent to the disease by the year 2003, with children below 15 years accounting for one in seven new global HIV infections and one in six global AIDS-related deaths. There are an estimated 0.17 million HIV+ children under 15 years in India (ibid.: 569). With regard to India's rural areas, home to 73 per cent of the country's population, studies show that at least in some areas HIV has become common with prevalence rates being higher than that in urban areas (Correa and Gisselquist 2005: 1; Verma and Roy 2002: 78).[8]

Gender is acknowledged as an inextricable part of the HIV/AIDS equation, with there being much talk of feminization of the epidemic (Falleiro and Noronha 2012; Medhini et al. 2007a: 449; Pradhan and Sundar 2006). Young women are disproportionately vulnerable to infection, with elderly women and young girls being disproportionately affected by the burden of caregiving (Medhini et al. 2007a: 449; Prasad 2008). Studies have shown that 90 per cent of India's HIV+ women have only one partner and are not involved in high-risk behaviour (UNFPA 2005, in Medhini et al. 2007a: 454). According to UNAIDS and WHO, over 38 per cent of the HIV+ people are women,[9] with the global rate of infected women rising in recent times to 50 per cent as per UNAIDS figures (A. Gandhi, in HRLN 2008: 91). Among youth, the gender gap is heightened with 75 per cent of all young PLWH being females (Medhini et al. 2007a: 448).

Women are biologically, epidemiologically and socially more vulnerable to HIV infection than men (Dixit 2005: 73–76; WHO 1995: 15). The peak age at which women are likely to report themselves HIV+ is about six years lower than men (Canning et al. 2006a: 11). In case of infected women, the majority have no other risk factor except than being married to their husbands (Medhini et al. 2007a: 448; Verma and Roy 2002: 79). Incidentally, most women complete their child bearing before falling ill, thereby leading to rise in the number of orphans.[10] As per WHO estimates about 2.2 million HIV+ women across the world give birth each year (Mascarenhas 2006: 13). In Goa 47.3 per cent of the HIV+ females in 2009 belonged to the age group of 15–34 years (GSACS 2009: 17).

In India, while in 83–85 per cent of the reported cases the HIV infection has been acquired through the sexual route, in 2.2–4 per cent it was through contaminated blood/blood product transfusion,

2.2–4 per cent through sharing of injection equipment during drug use, with perinatal transmission accounting for another 2–3.8 per cent of the cases. Incidentally, in 6.8–7 per cent of the cases the history of transmission is not available (Panda et al. 2002: 19; GSACS 2009: 9); with one possible cause of these *nosocomial* or unexplained cases being blood exposures in health care and cosmetic services (Correa and Gisselquist 2005).

The HIV/AIDS epidemic usually moves from high-risk groups such as commercial sex workers (CSWs) and drug users, to bridge populations like clients of CSWs, persons with sexually transmitted disease/infection (STD/STI) and partners of drug users, followed by the general population; with there being a time lag of about 3–5 years between the shift from one group to the other (Joshi 2000: 27). While people affected by HIV/AIDS have their rights violated, those who have their rights violated— including women, children, CSWs, drug addicts and those living in poverty—are vulnerable to the risk of HIV infection (WCC 2002: 73). Incidentally and additionally, the HIV/AIDS epidemic is not randomly distributed; it is clustered in households (HHs), geographically and occupationally, with the virus moving when people, especially those single, move (Reid 2000c: 782).

Economics provides a firm base for studying the pattern of spread of HIV; this is particularly the case under the hypothesis that HIV is not spread randomly like most other illnesses, but that it is instead spread via purposeful behaviour that has a strong economic foundation (Mahal and Rao 2005: 593). Some often cited economic causes of HIV/AIDS, with economic deprivation being the primary contributor and common factor, are: (i) poverty and low economic status; (ii) prostitution; (iii) gender inequalities; (iv) mobility/migration of population; (v) urbanization; (vi) food scarcity/insecurity; and (vii) economic inequality. Incidentally, it is not only the poorer or marginalized sections that are prone to HIV infections; those from the higher socio-economic status too have had high infection rates as studies of some African countries have revealed (Rao 2000b: 495), with possible causes being: (a) high education/income making it easy to support/attract additional commercial/casual sex partners; and (b) those with more income/ education being likely to travel and have more opportunities for variety of sexual contacts (Israni 2001: 157; Ramakrishna et al. 2008: 386).

HIV/AIDS has far reaching consequences, with social, economic, medical, ethical, political, psychological and legal being just a few. The epidemic has often been associated with adverse public reactions, unlike reactions for other ailments like cancer, diabetes or heart diseases. Incidentally, these reactions besides shaping the behaviour of PLWHA also hinder the effectiveness of prevention efforts (Mawar et al. 2005: 472). Often the social stigma attached to HIV/AIDS does not get erased even post death (Kelly et al. 1996; Mawar and Paranjape 2002, both in Mawar et al. 2005: 472–473). The seriousness of the socio-economic impact of HIV/AIDS led to the setting up of NACO in 1992, with the vision to lead and catalyse an expanded response to the HIV/AIDS problem in order to contain its spread, reduce people's vulnerability and promote care within an enabling environment (Joshi 2000: 28–29).

Adverse economic fallouts of HIV/AIDS are experienced at the micro/individual/HH, macro/national and sectoral levels. HIV/AIDS has been found contributing to rise in (in)direct costs and poverty, diversion of funds from development, repayment problems vis-à-vis international debts and strain on fiscal budgets of developing countries. According to a study conducted by National Council of Applied Economic Research (NCAER) backed by NACO and UNDP, in the absence of remedial policy, the HIV epidemic in India from 2002–2003 to 2015–2016, was likely to push up health spending by HHs and the state, thereby eating into savings, crowding-out investment and hitting growth. The study forecast that economic growth and GDP per capita would decline by 0.86 and 0.55 percentage points respectively over the period; besides slowing the growth of labour supply, lowering labour productivity and cutting into non-food expenditures of HHs due to rise in health expenditures (Ojha and Pradhan 2006: xxi; Sharma and Baxi 2007: 12). It has been claimed that by not considering HIV/ AIDS as an humanitarian activity alone and by focusing instead administrative resources and expenditure in checking the growth of HIV/AIDS, could boost India's economic growth by 1 per cent per annum till the year 2016 (see Ojha and Pradhan 2006: xxi).[11]

AIDS epidemic hits harder the sectors that use unskilled labour intensively. The total loss of value added in terms of real GDP on account of HIV/AIDS for the year 2015–2016 was estimated at 9.89 per cent, with manufacturing and tourism taking the hardest hit (Ojha and Pradhan 2006: xx). HIV/AIDS has two major effects on industry, the first on the workforce through increase in absenteeism, recruitment and training costs, funeral costs, lost knowledge, reduced morale, etc; and the second through reduction in consumer base, especially in regions with high HIV prevalence where reallocation of resources takes place in favour of health care in comparison to other sectors (ibid.: 4–5). Besides manufacturing and tourism, the other major sectors experiencing the adverse impact of HIV/AIDS the world over have been transport, health, agriculture and education. To list a few additional fallouts of HIV/AIDS, it has been found that it hits harder the smaller production units, leads to fall in output produced, contributes to diversion from commercial/cash crop to food crop cultivation, decrease in non-farm income, shift to less labour-intensive cash crops, decline in area cultivated and less animal husbandry.

Bloom and Mahal (1997) contend that economic costs of AIDS will be felt not by nations but by communities and HHs (in Kadiyala and Barnett 2004: 1891). The fallouts of HIV/AIDS commence immediately after an infected HH member becomes prone to HIV related infections and complications. HIV/AIDS necessitates steps that need to be taken to reorganize division of labour within HHs so as to reallocate productive tasks to non-infected members (Reid 2000a: 21). The areas of economic impact of HIV/AIDS at the individual/HH level, particularly on those from the poorer brackets on account of weaker resilience, include employment,[12] education,[13] consumption/savings and borrowings. A NACO, UNDP and NCAER study indicated that HH incomes would come down especially for rural non-agricultural self-employed, followed by rural agricultural labour, rural non-agricultural labour, rural agricultural self-employed and urban casual labour, since all these are unskilled labour providers—the group worst hit by HIV.[14] Booysen (2003) found that over time HHs with HIV+ members were relatively more likely to experience income variations and chronic poverty; with HIV related consequences such as mortality, morbidity and orphaning playing a role in explaining socio-economic mobility of HHs (in Werker et al. 2007: 26).

At the HH level, where gender-biases against females are anything but rare, the most obvious impact of HIV/AIDS is the increased spending on treatment and care (Falleiro and Noronha 2011; 2012). Incidentally, though treatment is of utmost essence the overwhelming majority of PLWHA in India are unable to avail, access or afford the same. While studies generally reveal insignificant support from social security or insurance, with there being high dependence on public hospitals and NGOs; evidence suggests that employers discriminate against HIV+ employees when it comes to benefits related with illness (see Canning et al. 2006a: 13; 2006b). Bloom and Mahal (1996) and Bloom and Glied (1993) estimated the ratio of treatment costs to per capita income to be 2.2 in India, with the treatment costs not including the cost of ARV drugs (in Ojha and Pradhan 2006: 2; see also ADB 2004: 58; Mahal and Rao 2005: 583). In addition to high medical expenses, HIV/AIDS contributes to a fall in HH income, irrespective of whether the HIV infected member is dead or alive, besides creating other hardships which can have a negative impact on the future well-being of HHs, including HH members having lower long-term accumulations of human capital, be it in terms of health or education (Ojha and Pradhan 2006: 3).

As time passes, HIV/AIDS becomes increasingly concentrated among poor populations;[15] while the wealthy countries and rich individuals learn to protect themselves and have the resources to make HIV/AIDS into a chronic but not deadly disease, the poor nations and poverty stricken majority remain vulnerable (Bertozzi et al. 2001). The serious nature of HIV/AIDS made world leaders during the United Nations Millennium Summit in September 2000 to agree upon as one of the eight specific and measurable development goals, the Millennium Development Goals (MDG), the halting and reversing the spread of HIV/AIDS (IMF 2005).

Notes

1. Both were awarded the 2008 Nobel Prize in medicine for their discovery; an award shared with Harald zur Hausen who studied the cause of cervical cancer.
2. See 'AIDS numbers rising across the world'. *The Times of India (TOI)*, Mumbai, 23 November 2006, 11.
3. See 'One out of every 100 adults is HIV-positive'. *TOI*, Mumbai, 7 June 2007, 7.
4. Number of cases in relation to total population.
5. Incidentally, while *concentrated epidemic* can also refer to situations where there is concentration of infection among high-risk groups, *general epidemic* can refer to situations where there is spread of infection among the general population. There is no proper agreement as to the factors responsible for the differences between the two (Correa et al. 2008: 2).
6. See 'Dramatic fall in HIV cases, but war is on: NACO'. *The Economic Times (ET)* 7 July 2007.
7. See 'Ribbon of Solidarity'. *TOI* 1 December 2008, 7.
8. See also 'AIDS a major problem despite dropping figures'. *TOI* 29 November 2007, 6.
9. See Sinha (2006b).
10. HIV/AIDS Forum: Impact of the HIV/AIDS epidemic; at: http://www.indianngos.com/issue/hiv/resources/impact.htm, accessed July 2007.
11. See also 'AIDS to Knock 0.9% off GDP'. *ET* 21 July 2006, 1.
12. To include loss of income/employment for the infected person/caregiver/non-infected member due to death/leave/absence from work or lack of employment; reduced employability because of sickness/discrimination; high workforce participation rate among children/elderly, etc.
13. Typical fallouts include absenteeism, withdrawal from school/high drop-out rate due to illness, cost of education, employment seeking role for children, caregiving role for children, etc.
14. See 'AIDS to Knock 0.9% off GDP' *ET* 21 July 2006, 1.
15. ADB (2004: 3); Dixit (2005: 142); Kadiyala and Barnett (2004: 1891); Mahal and Rao (2005: 593); Medhini et al. (2007b: 1088); Narain (2004: 29); UNAIDS (2006: 84–85), etc., have all made references to the disproportionate impact of HIV/AIDS on poorer HHs and/or how HIV/AIDS is usually concentrated among those from the marginalized and poorer economic segments.

2

Income and Employment

Employment is not only an economic necessity but also an important source of dignity and self esteem, as well as a medium for daily social interaction with co-workers (Medhini et al. 2007a: 153).

HIV/AIDS places new demands on HH resources and reduces the time that adults can spend on income-generating activities (Dixit 2005: 110). The present chapter highlights the varied nature of fallouts of HIV/AIDS on the income and employment of individuals and HHs. To put things in proper perspective, findings of the comparative analyses involving the matched sample of non-HIV/AIDS HHs has also been presented herein. The chapter additionally reveals how affected HHs cope up with the dilemma of falling income and rising expenditure.

2.1 General

One of the major economic consequences of HIV/AIDS is its adverse impact on income and employment pertaining to HHs since it primarily affects individuals from the economically productive age group. Reasons attributed to the loss of income and employment include among others: (i) premature death, (ii) currently working HIV+ individuals forced to take leave or be absent from work due to ill health and (iii) employed caregivers having to remain absent from work to look after the HIV+ members (see Pradhan et al. 2006).

To begin the study highlights with a brief mention of the nature of occupation of the sample respondents/HHs and their educational qualifications (see Appendix I: Table AI.iii) since it has a bearing on income and employment, most of the HH heads of both the samples (that is, HIV/AIDS and non-HIV/AIDS HHs) were employed in construction and related work, were skilled/ semi-skilled/non-agricultural labourers, or were in 'service'. While numbers of the retired/pensioners were almost the same in both the samples, there were more domestic servants (10 per cent) and those who could not work due to sickness (20.5 per cent) in the HIV/AIDS HHs sample as compared to those in the control group (that is, non-HIV/AIDS HHs) where the figures were 4.5 and 1 per cent respectively.

With regard to educational profile of the HH heads, the two samples were more or less identical, with illiterate HH heads constituting about 36 per cent of the total (see Appendix I: Table AI.ii). If one considers the highest level of occupation (in terms of nature of work, designation and/or monetary earnings) and educational qualifications that any HH member had, excluding the HH head[1] (see Appendix I: Table AI.iv): *firstly*, almost in 35 per cent HHs in both samples the better occupation was held by a member other than the HH head;[2] and *secondly*, while in HIV/AIDS HHs 54 per cent of the HH heads had relatively superior educational qualifications as compared to other HH members, in case of non-HIV/AIDS HHs the figure was lower at 33.5 per cent. The second of the above is an indicator, as confirmed through field interactions, of HIV/AIDS having the tendency of depriving younger HH members of affected HHs from higher education.[3] Incidentally, not having sufficient/higher education can deprive HH member's better employment and higher earnings, present as well as future.

Of the two samples, the HIV/AIDS HHs sample had fewer HH members as well as fewer working and thus earning members (see Table 2.1i). While 30.90 per cent of the members of HIV/ AIDS HHs were working, the figure was higher at 40.34 per cent for non-HIV/AIDS HHs. Loosely related to the dependency ratio, while the number of non-working members in HIV/AIDS HHs

Table 2.1i

Households sample profile vis-à-vis annual HH income

	HIV/AIDS HHs	Non-HIV/AIDS HHs
Total no. of HHs	**200**	**200**
Total HH members	**754** *(Mean:3.77;SD:1.86)*	*895 (Mean: 4.48; SD:1.50)*
Number of working members	**233***(Mean:1.17; SD: 0.86)*	*361(Mean: 1.81; SD: 0.89)*
No. of non-working members	**521** *(Mean:2.61;SD: 1.65)*	*534 (Mean:2.67; SD: 1.40)*
Wage income		
No. of HHs where wage income per annum is **nil**	19	2
Average HH wage income per annum per HH	₹58,025 (SD: 78611)	₹1,04,990 (SD: 76385)
Average wage income per HH member per annum	₹15,391	₹23,464
Average annual wage income per working member	₹49,807	₹58,172
No. of HHs having **nil** wage **and nil** non-wage income p.a.*	10	0
Non-wage income		
No. of HHs having non-wage income excl. interest	50	25
No. of HHs with **nil** non-wage income p.a. (excluding interest)	150	175
No. of HHs with **nil** non-wage income; but with interest earnings	38	138
No. of HHs with interest (exclusively or with other non-wage incomes)	29	161
No. of HHs with **nil** non-wage income p.a.(and **nil** interest earnings)	112	37
Total non-wage income per HH excluding interest earnings	₹5,111 (SD: 14321)	₹2,294 (SD: 9944)

(Table 2.1i Continued)

(Table 2.1i Continued)

	HIV/AIDS HHs	Non-HIV/AIDS HHs
Total HH income per annum		
Average total HH income per annum (per HH)	₹63,126 (SD: 81220)	₹1,07,280 (SD: 76750)
Average income per HH member per annum (approx/rounded-up)	₹16,750	₹23,800

Source: Author's field work.
Note: *Not even interest.

was about 2.24 times that of working members, it was relatively better at about 1.48 in case of non-HIV/AIDS HHs. If we consider dependency in terms of total population vis-à-vis total number of earners (Pradhan et al. 2006: 42), the ratio is 3.24 and 2.48 in HIV/AIDS and non-HIV/AIDS HHs' samples respectively. We can thus conclude that there were relatively more dependants in HIV/AIDS HHs.[4] This situation can only get worse; in Botswana, it was estimated that an income earner was likely to acquire an additional dependant over the next 10 years, with families in the poorest quartile to acquire an additional eight dependants on account of AIDS (UNAIDS 2006: 84; see also Greener 2004, in UNAIDS 2008: 23 and 170). To highlight the gravity of the situation of non-working/earning members in HIV/AIDS HHs from another viewpoint, 15.5 per cent HHs in the present study had currently no employed member; the corresponding figure for non-HIV/AIDS HHs was only 1 per cent.

HIV/AIDS HHs have generally fewer HH members. The primary reasons for the same are: (i) a number of members have already died of AIDS and (ii) in a number of instances the families have been isolated, with other family members staying separate ever since HIV detection.[5] Other studies have confirmed that AIDS related death to a bread-winner occasionally leads to HHs facing disbanding or dissolution (see Dixit 2005: 110; Gaigbe-Togbe and Weinberger 2003: 32). According to Pradhan et al. (2006: 43), the small size of HHs could be for reasons like PLWHA generally living in nuclear family and/or preferring not to have children. The size of working/earning members is fewer in HIV/AIDS HHs since a number of members are unable to work as a consequence of HIV/AIDS, for example, due to sickness or caregiving duties.

That HIV/AIDS has adverse implications on 'per HH wage income', 'per capita wage income' and 'per working member wage income' with all being substantially lower in HIV/AIDS HHs as compared to non-HIV/AIDS HHs can be seen in Table 2.1i. While the annual average wage income per HIV/AIDS HH is only about 0.55 times that of non-HIV/AIDS HHs, the average wage income per HIV/AIDS HH member per annum is about 0.66 times that of the control group. The per capita wage income per working/earning member in HIV/AIDS HHs which is proportionately 0.86 times that of non-HIV/AIDS HHs, is low on account of reasons like: (i) absenteeism due to sickness and/or caregiving; (ii) frequent changes in jobs, denying the benefit of increments and better earnings particularly in case of salaried individuals; (iii) in case of wage earners, full time work becomes part time work due to HIV/AIDS contributed weakness/indisposition, etc. Incidentally, while 19 (9.5 per cent) HIV/AIDS HHs had no wage income due to HIV/AIDS contributed reasons, the figure for non-HIV/AIDS HHs sample was only two (1 per cent). Likewise, while 10 (5 per cent) HIV/AIDS HHs had neither wage nor non-wage income during the last 12 months, the figure was nil for non-HIV/AIDS HHs. Reference to the 'dramatic' increase in number of destitute HHs, that is, those with no income earners, can be found also in Greener (2004, in UNAIDS 2006: 85).

With regard to annual non-wage HH income, except for the 'numbers' of HHs having non-wage income (excluding interest)[6] and the 'value' of total non-wage income per HH (excluding interest) where the relative figures were *very significantly* higher and better for HIV/AIDS HHs; the figures in general for non-HIV/AIDS HHs were far superior to those of HIV/AIDS HHs. For instance, while there were 161 (80.5 per cent) non-HIV/AIDS HHs enjoying interest earnings, exclusively or along with other non-wage earnings, the corresponding number was only 29 (14.5 per cent) HIV/AIDS HHs.

Also, while 37 (18.5 per cent) non-HIV/AIDS HHs had nil non-wage earnings (including nil interest), the figure was much higher in case of HIV/AIDS HHs at 112 (56 per cent). Incidentally, the numbers of HIV/AIDS HHs with non-wage income (excluding interest) were higher and so also the per HH non-wage income (excluding interest), since unlike their non-HIV/AIDS counterparts, there were more widows, many of who were receiving Government of Goa provided pension on account of death of their husbands, majority of who died of AIDS.[7] That widow's pension plays an important role in HIV/AIDS HHs can be seen by the *quite significant* difference existing in the total annual non-wage income (excluding interest) for the entire HIV/AIDS HHs sample based on gender of the HH head, with the mean annual non-wage income being about ₹7,867 for female-headed HHs and ₹3,156 for male-headed HHs.

With reference to the total HH income—wage and non-wage combined—the size of the HIV/AIDS HHs income is 0.59 times the size of their counterparts, with the average annual income per HH member being 0.70 times. As can be seen from Table 2.1i, the per capita annual income per HIV/AIDS HH member is ₹16,750 as compared to ₹23,800 in case of non-HIV/AIDS HH members; this despite family size being relatively smaller in the former. Fall in levels of per capita and HH incomes due to HIV/AIDS have also been recorded by other studies; for instance a study in Botswana, found that HIV results in a decline in per capita HH income by 10 per cent, with average income losses being almost twice as high for HHs in the lowest income level (see UNAIDS 2008: 162).

The mean total annual income per HH between the two samples' was found to be different from each other by an amount of about ₹44,154 (see Table 2.1i). Statistical testing has affirmed the differences to be *highly significant* in nature. Incidentally, tests also show that there was *highly significant* difference in total annual HH income based on gender of the HH heads in both samples' to the disadvantage of female-headed HHs. While mean total annual HH income for male-headed and female-headed HIV/AIDS HHs was ₹76,982 (SD: 95078) and ₹43,593 (SD: 50606) respectively; the corresponding figures were ₹1,14,310 (SD: 74113) and ₹85,031 (SD: 81416) respectively in case of the non-HIV/AIDS HHs sample.

2.2 Death of an HIV/AIDS Member

One important socio-economic impact of an AIDS related death is the loss of HH labour production; the production loss was estimated to be close to 50 per cent, leading to about 47 per cent loss in the HH income (Gaigbe-Togbe and Weinberger 2003: 32). Needless to say, an adult who dies prematurely generally produces less over the life cycle than one who does not. With reference to the present study, among the 200 HIV/AIDS HHs, 77 (38.5 per cent) HHs experienced at least one death of an AIDS member. Of those who died with AIDS, 70 members (from 70 HHs), used to be working members; 33 working at the time of death and 37 working earlier before HIV/AIDS made them to quit (see Table 2.2i). The average number of months (since they left work) for the 37 members who left their job before death was 12.22 months (SD: 11.89); with some having lost their employment/earnings and thus becoming economically unproductive for as high as five years (see Table 2.2ii). Incidentally, as mentioned in the earlier section, the death of an earning member to AIDS tends to reduce the economic viability of the HH, with some HHs facing the possibility of disbanding or dissolution (see also Nielsen and Melgaard 2004: 45). A study of rural South Africa (Hosegood et al. 2003) found HHs experiencing at least one AIDS death during the year were nearly thrice likely to dissolve compared to other HHs (in Gaigbe-Togbe and Weinberger 2003: 32).[8] That loss of HH members can lead to dissolution/disbanding has been found by the present study as well. While there were 22 (11 per cent) single-person HIV/AIDS sample HHs, there was only one (0.5 per cent) non-HIV/AIDS HH. This is in sharp contrast to the 'one member HHs' figures for Goa as provided by Census of India (2001) which stands at 5.8 per cent and 5.7 per cent for rural and urban areas respectively.

Only seven of the 77 members who died of AIDS, never worked; among who were five minors and one housewife. Over 57 per cent of the dead members had earnings in the range of ₹2,001–5,000 per month, with the figure becoming about 65 per cent, if we exclude non-working members and two earning members whose earnings are unknown. If we include the dead members whose earnings were

Table 2.2i

Employment status, income-slabs and number of years since death of dead AIDS HH members

	Frequency	Per cent figures for entire sample	Per cent figures for only those dead
Employment status of the dead AIDS members			
Yes—employed at the time of death	33	16.5	42.9
Yes—but **not** at time of death but earlier*	37	18.5	48.1
Never employed#	7	3.5	9.1
Total—HHs of dead members	77	38.5	100
Others—that is, those who did not die	123	61.5	
Income slabs of the dead AIDS members			
Never employed	7	3.5	9.1
Up to ₹1,000	4^	2	5.2
₹1,001–2,000	12	6	15.6
₹2,001–3,500	27	13.5	35.1
₹3,501–5,000	17	8.5	22.1
₹5,001–7,500	3	1.5	3.9
₹7,501–10,000	3	1.5	3.9
₹10,001–20,000	2	1	2.6
Above ₹20,000	2	1	2.6
Total—HHs of dead members	77	38.5	100
Others—that is, those who did not die	123	61.5	
Number of years back the AIDS members died			
Below 2 years	12	6	15.6
2–5 years	35	17.5	45.5
5–10 years	23	11.5	29.9
Above 10 years	7	3.5	9.1
Total —HHs of dead members	77	38.5	100
Others—that is, those who did not die	123	61.5	
Total of all HHs	200	100	

Source: Author's field work.
Notes: *Had to give up job due to HIV/AIDS contributed sickness.
#Includes five minors, one housewife and a youth in the early twenties who never got an opportunity to work.
^Includes the two whose earnings are unknown.

Table 2.2ii

Details pertaining to the dead AIDS members

	Total members	Min.	Max.	Mean	SD
Number of months before dying left job*	37	1	60	12.22	11.9
Earnings lost per person per month (₹)	77	00	80,000	4,673#	9455.6
Earnings lost per dead working AIDS HH member (₹)	68##	1,000	80,000	5,292	9904.4
Age of dead persons (years)	77	2	60	33.56	11.1
Number of months suffering before death	77	1	60	11.12	12.4
Expenses incurred on funeral (₹)	77	1^^	25,000	4,898^	5158.3
Expenses incurred on funeral (where expense details are known) (₹)	54	500	25,000	6,983	4828.8

Source: Author's field work.

Notes: *Meant for those who were employed earlier but not at the time of death.
#Mean earnings per month shown are of all dead members taken together.
##These figures exclude the seven non-earning and two earning members whose earnings prior to death are unknown.
^This figure represents mean funeral expenses of all dead taken together (including 23, whose funeral expenses were unknown and/or whose expenditure was entirely sponsored by relations outside the HH).
^^Re. 1 stands for cases where funeral expenses were unknown or were fully sponsored by externals (that is, non-HH members).

over ₹5,000 per month, almost 80 per cent of the HHs having at least one dead earning AIDS member have lost substantial amounts of HH incomes; substantial considering the socio-cultural-economic background of the HHs, prevailing educational qualifications, expenditure patterns, etc. The mean earnings lost per dead member were ₹4,673, or ₹5,292 if we consider only the working members whose earnings are known (see Table 2.2ii). On a per annum basis, the income lost per HH is over ₹63,500; a figure which happens to be higher than the annual total HH income of 73 per cent sample HHs.

Notwithstanding the losses of income cited, in reality the same are much bigger since they add-up over the years post death. In Ivory Coast, urban HHs that lost at least one member to AIDS, have seen their income drop by 52–67 per cent, with expenditures soaring four fold.[9] It was found in South Africa that HHs that experienced illness or death were more than twice likely to be poor than non-affected HHs, besides being likely to experience long-term poverty as well (Dixit 2005: 142). To make matters worse these sources of income have ceased for many years for a large number of HHs (see Table 2.2i), with almost 30 per cent and 9 per cent of the dead earning AIDS members of the present study, having died between '5 and 10 years' and 'above 10 years' earlier, respectively. Incidentally, studies in Tanzania found PLWHA experiencing on an average 12 months of deteriorating health before death (Bollinger et al. 1999; Beegle 2003, in UNAIDS 2008: 162). With regard to the present study, if one considers all earning members, the corresponding figure becomes 11.12 months (see Table 2.2ii). Needless to say, this figure has an adverse bearing not only on HH income but also on HH expenditure as well.

That death caused by AIDS to working members can have a severe adverse economic bearing on the HHs' present and future can be additionally gauged by the fact that an overwhelming majority of the dead members were in the economically productive age groups, with about 74 per cent being within 18–40 years and almost 90 per cent within 18–50 years. If we exclude the minors who died at very young age, the said figures rise even higher to 81.4 per cent and 98.6 per cent respectively (see Appendix II: Table AII.i). The mean age of dead members as shown in Table 2.2ii was 33.56 years (SD: 11.07). In the context of 'demographic gift' of Bloom and Williamson (1998), it is said that death (and morbidity) caused by HIV/AIDS among those in prime working ages can cause a 'reverse demographic gift', thereby adversely affecting growth[10] (Mahal and Rao 2005: 590). As Dixon et al. (2001) reiterate, AIDS which predominantly affects adults, could result in severe economic effects in the context of decreasing human capital and economic growth (in Werker et al. 2007: 2). The economic impact of high mortality rate especially among working age group members becomes all the more serious because of the huge private and public investments that have already been made on the same (World Bank 2003: 5). Majority of the dead members in the present study were skilled/semi-skilled/non-agricultural workers, construction (and related) workers, and truck/non-truck drivers/transport workers; with the remaining being mostly in private/government service or having petty business/small shops (see Appendix II: Table AII.i).

Loss of employment on account of AIDS contributed death is of no economic gain to HHs, possibly (as may be argued by a few) barring the sole exception that it could have reduced the high medical expenditures often linked with the treatment of OIs associated with HIV/AIDS. However, despite the same it needs to be reiterated that besides every adult who dies of AIDS leaving behind dependent HH members, in economic terms the indirect costs due to loss of productivity exceed health care costs; a study in Thailand indicated that health care cost for an AIDS patient was US$1,500 compared to the indirect cost to the economy of US$22,000 in case of death (Rao 2000b: 495). In India and Sri Lanka, lifetime earnings lost due to AIDS related death were estimated to be more than 10 times the annual treatment expenses of AIDS (Mahal and Rao 2005: 584). Under conservative assumptions of working life span and discount rates, the loss in lifetime earnings as shared by Bloom and Mahal (1996) were said to be 3.5 times the annual costs of treatment of AIDS (in Ojha and Pradhan 2006: 2).

Of the 70 HHs from where earning members died of AIDS, only three got benefit of Provident Fund (PF), with two getting insurance and two pension; the remaining got neither financial assistance nor employment for surviving HH members. Incidentally, for those who got the financial benefit, much of the same went towards meeting funeral expenses, with very little remaining for HH support. Related to funeral expenses, the average expenses for the dead members were ₹4,898 for all members taken together (even if expenditure details were unknown); and ₹6,983 for the 54 members whose funeral expenditure details were known (Table 2.2ii). In the case of 26 HHs/dead AIDS members, the funeral expenses were above the ₹6,983 average; with the expenses being as high as ₹25,000. Needless to say, funeral expenses have drained much more of the scarce resources of HHs which lost two or more members to AIDS.

The present study revealed that death of earning AIDS members was witnessed primarily in female-headed HHs (61 of the 77 HHs which experienced death were female-headed); with statistical tests showing the association to be *very significant*. Unsurprisingly, tests also showed *very significant* difference in earnings (lost) of dead AIDS earning members in HIV/AIDS HHs based on gender of the HH head. On a related note, *significant* difference was found in the total annual HH income in HIV/AIDS HHs based on gender of the HH head where death of AIDS members took place. Female-headed HHs have significant hardships to face since the dead members were usually male members; often the male-head and spouse of the present female-head herself (see also Dixit 2005: 110–111 and 142). The statement that female-headed HHs face significant hardships on the death of earning AIDS member has been made under the assumption that death leads to loss of income, which as Table 2.6.3ii (Section 2.6.3) reveals is a substantial amount.[11]

Notwithstanding the huge loss of HH income due to death of AIDS earning members as highlighted, the loss becomes far worse when: (i) the dead member was the only earning member, and (ii) there were two or more earning members in the HH who died of AIDS.

2.3 Income and Employment of the HIV+ Respondents[12]

2.3.1 Previous and Present Employment

Of the 200 HIV+ sample respondents, only 9 per cent never worked; with 47 per cent who worked at the time of HIV detection, working presently as well (Table 2.3.1i). While 30 per cent who were working earlier were currently not working due to HIV/AIDS; 11 per cent of those not working earlier were presently working to make up for the fall in HH income and to meet rising expenses (particularly medical) due to HIV/AIDS to self or other HH members. Incidentally, 3 per cent respondents who were neither working at the time of HIV detection nor are presently working, were working in between, but had to give up the job due to inability and indisposition on account of HIV/AIDS.[13]

Table 2.3.1i

Past and present employment status of the HIV+ respondents*

	Frequency	Per cent
Working earlier, working now	94	47
Working earlier, not working now	60	30
Not working earlier, working now	22	11
Not working earlier, not working now—'never worked'	18	9
Not working earlier, not working now—'worked in between'	6	3
Total	**200**	**100**

Source: Author's field work.
Note: *At the time of detection of HIV.

As in Table 2.3.1ii, 53 per cent of the total sample respondents had to change or quit their job after knowing about their HIV+ status. If we exclude those who were not employed at the time, the figure becomes even higher at almost 69 per cent. Of these, 57.5 per cent had to change or quit the job on account of being too ill to work, with another 14.2 per cent getting dismissed from work; dismissed not because of inability to work, but because of the stigma attached to those with HIV infection (Table 2.3.1iii). Incidentally, in cases of dismissal from service (despite being fit for work) the total size of earnings lost could be greater than those compared to if one had to leave the job due to being too ill to work, since the time over which the HH is without income would be longer. It needs to be added that leaving aside dismissal from service and the role played by discrimination, the poor health contributed

Table 2.3.1ii

'Change in job' status of HIV+ respondent after HIV detection

	Frequency	Per cent
Changed job	106	53
Did not change job	48	24
Not employed at the time	46	23
Total	**200**	**100**

Source: Author's field work.

Table 2.3 1iii

Reasons for leaving job, whether received benefits and number of times changed jobs

	Frequency	% of total sample HHs	% of those who had to leave job
Reason for leaving the job			
Too ill to work	61	30.5	57.5
Dismissed from work	15	7.5	14.2
Took voluntary retirement	3	1.5	2.8
Discrimination at workplace	1	.5	.9
Others	26	13	24.5
Sub-total	*106*	*53*	*100*
Those not employed at time of HIV detection and who did not have to leave the job	94	47	
Whether received benefits at the time of leaving the job			
No benefit	94	47	88.7
Provident Fund (PF)	5	2.5	4.7
Compensation	5	2.5	4.7
N.A. (self-employed/own business)	1	.5	.9
Others	1	.5	.9
Sub-total	*106*	*53*	*100*
Those not employed at time of HIV detection and who did not have to leave the job	94	47	
Number of times changed job after detection of HIV+ status			
1 time	25	12.5	23.6
2 times	13	6.5	12.3
3 times	2	1	1.9
4 times	4	2	3.8
5 to 11 times	5	2.5	4.6
12 times	1	.5	.9
Did not take up job again	56	28	52.8
Sub-total	*106*	*53*	*100*
Those not employed at time of HIV detection and who did not have to leave the job	94	47	
Total	**200**	**100**	

Source: Author's field work.

by HIV/AIDS itself, is the main factor responsible for the loss of employment/income. In the context of discrimination though, things on the employment front can only worsen if one adds the role played by potential discrimination, that is, if HIV+ employees inform their employers about their status. Discrimination can be economically harmful as it excludes qualified and able workers from the labour force and unnecessarily increases the burden on the social security system, besides making those infected to unnecessarily change jobs (Medhini et al. 2007a: 153 and 161). Fear of stigma/discrimination can even encourage individuals to ignore their HIV status, with denial being a natural ally of discrimination (Jain 2008a: 11). Incidentally, pertaining to the present study, of those who had to change their job after knowing their HIV+ status, while the majority of 52.8 per cent never worked again, most of the remaining changed their job on one or two occasions, with one respondent changing as high as 12 times.

Close to 89 per cent of those who changed/quit their job received neither financial compensation nor any other benefit from their employers at the time of leaving. Of those who received compensation, ranging from a paltry ₹500 to a high of ₹3,00,000, the mean amount received was ₹49,318 (Table 2.3.1iv). One reason for the majority not getting compensation was that most[14] were employed in the private unorganized sector, with 22 being illiterate.

Pertaining to those currently working, with regard to certain occupations there were a few noticeable shifts in the types of jobs in which the respondents were employed (see Table 2.3.1v). While there was a fall in number of agricultural and skilled/semi-skilled/non-agricultural labourers (also in Pradhan et al. 2006: xxi), there

Table 2.3.1iv

Amount received by those who got financial compensation at the time of leaving the job

	No. of individuals/ HHs	Min. (₹)	Max. (₹)	Mean (₹)	SD
Amount received at the time of leaving job	11	500	3,00,000	49,318	86817

Source: Author's field work.

Table 2.3.1v

Notable job changes: Past and present*

Nature of job	Earlier number (time of HIV detection)	Present number
Agricultural labour	3	0
Skilled/semi-skilled/non-agricultural labour	30	21
Services	32	39
Petty business/small shop	3	9
Domestic servant	20	23
Housewife	7	0

Source: Author's field work.
Notes: *At the time of HIV detection.

was a rise of those in service, petty business/small shops and domestic servants.

That HIV/AIDS has an adverse impact on agricultural workers has been brought out by a number of studies. Fox et al. (2004) on a study involving tea pluckers in Kenya showed the adverse impact of HIV/AIDS in terms of attendance, productivity and earning power; one of the findings was that tea pluckers who died of AIDS produced about one-third less tea in their last two years of life than healthy workers (Fox et al. 2003, in Gaigbe-Togbe and Weinberger 2003: 35). With regard to agricultural workers and/or agriculture in the context of the present study, leaving aside that there were no agricultural workers presently employed in HIV/AIDS HHs though there were at the time of HIV detection, that HIV/AIDS has some (in)direct adverse bearing can be seen through a comparative glance of the two study samples. While in non-HIV/AIDS HHs there were 13 agricultural labourers/cultivators as HH heads, with 27 HHs owning livestock and 54 owning plots of land including those used for plantation, the corresponding figures were lower at only two, 11 and 37 respectively for HIV/AIDS HHs.

Comparable to the findings of the present study pertaining to agriculture/agricultural sector, other studies also found less ownership of assets, land, animals, etc. as a consequence of HIV/AIDS (see also Barnett and Blaikie 1992; Pradhan et al. 2006;

Verma et al. 2002). While it is possible that lack of assets in HIV/ AIDS HHs could be an indication of the poverty levels ante-HIV infection, the present study found that HIV/AIDS is an important factor contributing to the fall in assets holdings of HHs (see also Nielsen and Melgaard 2004: 44). The present study revealed non-HIV/AIDS HHs currently owning more assets than HIV/AIDS HHs (see Appendix I: Table AI.vii). On an argumentative note, even if one assumes that lesser assets were owned by HIV/AIDS HHs on account of pre-existing poverty, while non-HIV/AIDS HHs have built up their assets over time despite similar (earlier) background as HIV/AIDS HHs, the latter were unable to do so due to dwindling incomes and rising expenses on account of the dreaded infection.

The present rise in service jobs and domestic servants as brought out by the present study (see Table 2.3.1v) can be directly attributed to the following: (i) in case of services jobs a number of HIV+ individuals have been provided employment by NGOs linked with HIV/AIDS; (ii) with regard to domestic servants, the rise in numbers is due to its appealing nature for many, especially females, due to reasons such as flexibility in work hours, availability of at least one free meal (helps reduce one's own HH food expenses), closeness to one's residence (saves transport expenses), unskilled nature of job (unqualified individuals can take up the job) and availability of free time (for taking care of one's HH, for caregiving or for resting if one is HIV+). Incidentally, the seven 'unpaid' housewives at the time of HIV detection were conspicuous by their absence, since they had presently taken up remunerative jobs themselves to supplement HH income.

With regard to income slabs of those working at the time of HIV detection, working presently, or both, there has been a significant rise in the number of unemployed and hence of those belonging to the 'nil' income bracket (Table 2.3.1vi). While there were 22 who were not earning earlier, the figure has gone up to 60 at present, with the percentage figures being 12.5 and 34.01 respectively. There is thus a rise in unemployment post HIV detection, the same of which was also noted by the NCAER/NACO/UNDP study which showed an increase in percentage of unemployed PLWHA from 3.61 per cent before test to 9.80 per cent after test

Table 2.3.1vi

Monthly income slabs of those employed at time of HIV detection and now

Per month income slabs of HIV+ respondents	No. of those employed at time of HIV detection	Per cent of those employed at time of HIV detection	No. of those presently employed	Per cent of those presently employed
Nil (not employed)	22	12.5	60	34.1
Up to ₹1,000	21	11.9	16	9.1
₹1,001–2,000	37	21	38	21.6
₹2,001–3,500	35	19.9	21	11.9
₹3,501–5,000	26	14.8	19	10.8
₹5,001–7,500	14	8	10	5.7
₹7,501–10,000	8	4.5	2	1.1
₹10,001–20,000	6	3.4	6	3.4
Above ₹20,000	7	4	4	2.3
Total	**176**	**100**	**176**	**100**

Source: Author's field work.

(Pradhan et al. 2006: xxi). With regard to the others presently working also, barring an inconsequential case where there was one extra individual in the ₹1,001–2,000 per month bracket, there were generally more individuals in each income slab for the earlier employment as compared to the present. The mean earnings at present[15] were also much lower at ₹2,856 per month as opposed to ₹4,694 at the time of HIV detection, despite there normally being a periodic increase in earnings over time (Table 2.3.1vii). Earnings which were as high as ₹75,000 per month earlier were only as high as ₹37,000 at present. In case of 51.1 per cent of the respondents who ever worked, the earnings have become lower now, with the earnings of 15.3 per cent not undergoing any change (Table 2.3.1viii).

The primary reasons for changes in present earnings as compared to the earlier ones are as follows: (i) *Earnings are higher now.* This happens mainly because of three reasons: firstly, some of those who were not working earlier are working at present and hence their income slab shifts from 'nil' to a positive bracket; secondly,

Table 2.3.1vii

Monthly income of the earlier and present employment of the HIV+ respondents

	No. of individuals	Min.(₹)	Max. (₹)	Mean (₹)	SD
Monthly income at time of HIV-detection	176	.00	75,000	4,694	8568
Monthly income now	176	.00	37,000	2,856	5092

Source: Author's field work.

Table 2.3.1viii

Nature of change in earnings from the time of HIV detection to present earnings

	Frequency	Per cent
Higher now	59	33.5
Lower now	90	51.1
No change	27	15.3
Total	**176**	**100**

Source: Author's field work.
Note:*These are based on actual earnings in absolute figures (and not on the basis of monthly income slabs).

those who have not changed their job, get their annual increase in earnings; and thirdly, in a number of cases members have taken additional jobs; (ii) *Earnings are lower now*. This primarily takes place because: firstly, some of those working earlier are presently not working, and hence they shift from positive income brackets to the 'nil' income bracket; secondly, there is often a cut in earnings due to absenteeism, non-availability of leave, inability to work full-time, etc.; and thirdly, even where another previously non-working HH member takes up temporarily the job of the HIV+ respondent due to the latter's indisposition, the earnings are lower due to inexperience, immaturity or inappropriate temperament to the task; (iii) *No change in earnings*. This happens despite number of years since HIV detection on account of the fact that while earnings go up periodically, the same are neutralized in the case of HIV+ salaried individuals due to salary cuts on account of increased absenteeism. In case of wage earners, while wage rates rise periodically, HIV+ individuals cannot always work as much as before; their hours of work per day or days of work per month get reduced. Higher prevailing wage rate thus gets offset with lesser working hours or days of work. As a consequence, the present net earnings remain the same as before. It will not be wrong to state in relative terms, keeping in mind the regular rise in cost of living, earnings of over 66 per cent of those employed were lower at present, than what they were at the time of HIV detection.

2.3.2 Present Employment

As mentioned earlier, 24 HIV+ respondents neither worked at the time of HIV detection nor were presently working. Of the remaining 176, while 60 (34.1 per cent) were currently not working, 116 (65.9 per cent) were, albeit with the unpleasant fact that the average earnings of about 52 per cent were lower than even the prevailing official minimum wage rate in Goa, which at the time was ₹103 per day.

Majority of those working (50.9 per cent) did not disclose their HIV+ status to their employers (Table 2.3.2i), with the figure going up to 64 per cent if we exclude the 24 respondents who were self-employed. In a study involving the state of Maharashtra, the figure of those not reporting their HIV+ status to their employers was 79 per cent (Pradhan and Sundar 2006: vi). With regard to the present study, over 83 per cent of those who did not disclose their status admitted of not doing so on account of the fear of losing their job, compounded with the fear of stigma and discrimination. On an encouraging note though, among those in the present study who reported their HIV+ status, none faced discrimination. Notwithstanding the same, although this is in contrast to an ILO study on HIV discrimination in India which found approximately 6 per cent HIV+ respondents reporting discrimination in the workplace (in Medhini et al. 2007a: 161), it is pertinent to note that the true extent of discrimination may have been a positive figure had the HIV+ status been revealed by all. Incidentally, of those who reported their status to the employers, 20 were provided

Table 2.3.2i

Employment, discrimination and employer-support of presently employed HIV+ respondents

	Frequency	Per cent (for concerned categories only)
Number of HIV+ respondents currently working		
Yes	116	65.9
No	60	34.1
Total	176	100
If currently working, does employer know of HIV+ status		
Yes	33	28.4
No	59	50.9
N.A. (Self employed)	24	20.7
Total	116	100
If employer does not know of status, reasons for not disclosing the same		
Social discrimination and isolation	6	10.17
Fear of losing the job	49	83.05
Lowered prestige	4	6.78
Total	59	100
If employer knows of HIV+ status, whether faced any type of discrimination		
Yes	0	0
No	33	100
Total	33	100
If employer knows of status, is there any support from employer		
Yes	28	84.85
No	5	15.15
Total	33	100
If employer gives support, nature of support provided		
Reimbursement of medical expenses	2	7.14
Paid leave	3	10.71
Flexibility in work hours	2	7.14
Others (nutritional support and/or combination of above)	21	75
Total	28	100

Source: Author's field work.

work by HIV/AIDS associated NGOs and it was primarily these NGOs which were the employers providing support to the HIV+ respondents in numerous ways, including provision of nutritional and/or medical support, paid leave, financial advances and flexibility of work hours. Among the remaining who reported their HIV+ status to the employers, four were domestic servants whose employers came to know of the status due to regular absenteeism, indisposition, weakness and/or frequent visits to clinics/hospitals; three were cab drivers whose employers were in no regular contact since they resided abroad; and the rest were primarily unskilled/ semi-skilled workers or employees in shops.

In the productive sector one immediate consequence of HIV/ AIDS is the high level of absenteeism due to being increasingly afflicted with AIDS related illnesses and for taking a longer time away from work for seeking treatment (Rao 2000b: 496). Findings of a study in Kenya substantiate the same, with even healthy workers not being spared because many, particularly women, take time-off to attend to the health needs of infected HH members who need care (ibid.). Fox et al. (2004: 321) highlight that during their last three years of life, tea pluckers who ultimately were terminated because of AIDS, were absent from work almost twice as often as other pluckers. That HIV/AIDS has an adverse bearing on employment and income due to absenteeism caused by illness can also be seen in the present study which points to a big number of 44.8 per cent currently working HIV+ respondents who lost income over the last one year due to the same (Table 2.3.2ii). To put things in perspective the corresponding figure was only 10.10 per cent for non-HIV/AIDS HHs. The mean number of days absent for all working members was 34.36 days for HIV/AIDS HHs, as against 3.47 for non-HIV/ AIDS HHs (Table 2.3.2iii). In another study Duraisamy et al. (2003) had estimated the average loss to be 43 days per HIV+ person in a six month period (in Mahal and Rao 2005: 584).

For those who were sick and lost income during the course of the last one year due to absence, while the average number of days of absence was 65.04 days for the HIV+ working/earning respondents, it was only 18.05 for working/earning members from non-HIV/ AIDS HHs. To compound matters, as a study in a sugar estate in

Table 2.3.2ii

Whether earning HH members lost income last year due to sickness-caused absenteeism

	HIV/AIDS HHs		Non-HIV/AIDS HHs	
	No. of cases	Per cent for respective categories	No. of cases	Per cent for respective categories
Yes	52	44.8	20	10.10
No	28	24.1	31	15.66
N.A. (never absent)	36	31	147	74.24
Total of those currently working	116	100	198	100

Source: Author's field work.

Table 2.3.2iii

Days of sickness-contributed absenteeism of those currently working

	HIV/AIDS HHs				Non-HIV/AIDS HHs			
	No. of HHs/ members	Min	Max	Mean	SD	No. of HHs/ members	Min	Max	Mean	SD
For all presently working members	116	0	210	34.36	44.2	198	0	45	3.47	7.8
For those absent and lost income	52	3	210	65.04	49.2	20	3	45	18.05	12.5
For those absent but did not lose income	28	2	60	21.57	13.9	31	2	30	10.48	7.1

Source: Author's field work.

Zambia revealed, besides AIDS contributing to significant man-hours lost, even on returning to work HIV+ workers could often not perform their duties satisfactorily (Rao 2000b: 496). With reference to the present study, among those who were absent but did not lose income, the figures were once again better for the control group. Incidentally, while 210 days was the maximum number of days of absence due to illness in case of the HIV/AIDS HHs sample, it was only 45 days for the non-HIV/AIDS HHs sample. It is pertinent to note that details of absence mentioned herein are only those related to absence from work due to illness.

Besides adversely affecting HHs, absenteeism (or death) on account of illness or caregiving for sick members can additionally cause organizational disruption, underutilization of installed capacity and use of temporary staff, all of which can affect the quality of products and services and lead to decline in productivity and profits. Additionally, HIV/AIDS caused illnesses/death can lead to disorganization among workers due to factors such as increased staff turnover, declining morale and loss of skills and knowledge gained from experience (Sharma 2006: 131). Dixit (2005: 105) indicates that the costs of absenteeism and reduced productivity could be higher than the costs of death itself.

Related to the number of days absent from work due to illness, is the amount of income lost due to absenteeism. While amount lost during the last 12 months in HIV/AIDS HHs was as high as ₹44,000, it was only ₹4,500 for non-HIV/AIDS HHs (Table 2.3.2iv). The mean earnings lost in the case of *only* those losing income due to the absence were ₹7,210 and ₹1,620 respectively for the two groups of HHs. With regard to *all* working members taken together, irrespective of whether they lost income or not, the mean earnings lost during the last year was a substantial ₹3,232 for HIV/AIDS HHs and a paltry ₹164 for non-HIV/AIDS HHs. Statistical tests conducted on all presently working/earning members showed that the income lost during the last 12 months on account of absence from work due to illness was *very significantly* different between the

Table 2.3.2iv

Income lost due to illness-caused absence during the last one year

	HIV/AIDS HHs				Non-HIV/AIDS HHs				
	N	Min	Max	Mean	SD	N	Min	Max	Mean	SD
For ONLY those presently working and have lost income (₹)	52	150	44,000	7,210	8611	20	150	4,500	1,620	1218
For ALL presently working members (₹)	116	00	44,000	3,232	6771	198	00	4,500	164	619

Source: Author's field work.

two samples. Incidentally, while Duraisamy et al. (2003) estimated mean income lost per HIV+ person was about ₹3000 for a six-month period (in Mahal and Rao 2005: 584), Pradhan et al. (2006: xxii) revealed that the amount lost due to leave/absence in the last one year was ₹3,736.

In fine, we can add that when an earning HIV+ person who was absent from work due to illness dies, not only the temporary loss of income becomes permanent, but funeral costs also add to the burden (Gaigbe-Togbe and Weinberger 2003: 29). Unfortunately, besides dipping into precious savings to meet needs, HHs get some costs adjusted by reducing investments in productive activities, such as withdrawing children from school to save expenses or increase HH labour (ibid.).

2.4 Income and Employment Pertaining to the Caregiver

One of the secondary fallouts of HIV/AIDS for HHs is the gradual shift of attention and engagement of members, from remunerative activities to caregiving duties. This is so because HIV/AIDS often necessitates the assistance, services and/or time of another individual—the caregiver (CG); and it is usually women who are most responsible for care of sick family members (Medhini et al. 2007b: 1090–1091; D'Cruz 2004: 17). According to Walker et al. (1995), criterion for caregiving is, dependence by one on another for any activity essential for daily living; caregiving is thus assistance provided to someone who is dependent on the same (in D'Cruz 2004: 12).

At the outset it needs to be remembered that most of the sample respondents of the present study belonged to HHs from the lower income brackets and hence having full time caregiving facility was a luxury that most could ill afford considering that able HH members were required to work to supplement HH income due to rising expenses and falling incomes. Caregiving wherever done was thus often only part-time. Table 2.4i shows that majority of the HHs (54.5 per cent) required a CG, either to take care of the

Table 2.4i

Need for a caregiver in the HH

	Frequency	Percentage
Yes, for self (available at least part-time basis or occasionally)	51	25.5
No	91	45.5
Yes, but nobody available	42	21
Yes—not for self but for spouse/HH member	16	8
Total	200	100

Source: Author's field work.

HIV+ respondent or other HIV+ members. However, despite the need for a CG, 21 per cent of the said HHs had to do without one.[16] The average number of months for which caregiving was required was 12.33 months (Table 2.4ii).

In HHs where there was the benefit of CGs, while in case of 53.8 per cent HHs it was the spouse who did the job; in case of 10.8 per cent each, it was the children or parents (Table 2.4iii).[17] Majority of the CGs (61.29 per cent), who happened to be HH members or close relatives of the HIV+ individuals, were presently employed; with the majority being skilled/semi-skilled/non-agricultural labourers

Table 2.4ii

Months since caregiving required, age of CGs and amounts lost due to caregiving

	No. of HHs	Min.	Max.	Mean	SD
If CG is required, whether available or not, since when (months)	109	1	72	12.33	15.1
If CG is HH member/relative age of the CG (years)	62	13	72	35.19	12.5
If CG is presently employed and has lost income due to caregiving, total amount lost last year (₹)	30	1/200#	15,000	2,695*	3029.4

Source: Author's field work.

Notes: #₹1 indicates that actual earnings of one CG are unknown. Of those earnings lost last year which are known the lowest amount was ₹200.

*Average for 30 individuals including one whose lost income information for the last year was unavailable; if we exclude the same, mean income lost by 29 CGs last year due to caregiving becomes about ₹2,788.

Table 2.4iii

Identity, employment, occupation and age of CGs and whether lost income due to caregiving

	Percentage figure for CGs only
If caregiving required and is provided for the identity of the CG	
Spouse	53.8
Children	10.8
Parents	10.8
Siblings	4.6
Other relatives	13.8
Care and support centre/home	1.5
Others	4.6
If CG is HH member/relation, whether employed at present	
Yes	61.29
No	38.71
Present occupation of CGs	
Construction	11.6
Skilled/semi-skilled/non-agricultural labour	30.2
Service (government/private)	14
Petty business/small shop	11.6
Other transport worker	2.3
Pensioner/retired	2.3
Domestic servant	18.6
Housewife	4.7
Student	4.7
If CG is HH member/relative, age of the CG	
Up to 18 years	9.7
18–30 years	24.2
31–50 years	56.5
51–60 years	4.8
Above 60 years	4.8
Did CG who is presently employed lose any income due to absence from work	
Yes	78.95
No	21.05
Total	100

Source: Author's field work.

and domestic servants at 30.2 and 18.6 per cent respectively. The study revealed that especially with regard to female HH members who double-up as CGs, being domestic servants to supplement income is a matter of choice, primarily due to the flexibility of work hours on account of caregiving at other times. Table 2.4iii also shows that 9.7 and 4.8 per cent of the CGs were minors and members aged above 60 years respectively. Incidentally, the youngest CG was aged 13 years and the oldest 72 years. Children, the least acknowledged CGs within the home, take the adult role especially in nuclear families when a parent dies and there is no one to look after the others, some of who themselves may be HIV+ (D'Cruz 2001; UNAIDS 2000c, 2001; UNAIDS/UNICEF/USAID 2002; all in D' Cruz 2004: 53). With regard to those above 60 years as CGs, it is not uncommon to have grandparents performing the role often on account of incapacity or death of parents due to HIV/AIDS (see also D'Cruz 2004: 55; Dixit 2005: 142; Pradhan and Sundar 2006: 35; Pradhan et al. 2006: 42; Singhal and Rogers 2006: 23). As Dixit (2005: 111) indicates, HIV/AIDS can lead to increase in multi-generational HHs without the middle income-generating one. Pertaining to the present study, majority (85.5 per cent) of the employed CGs who were HH members or relatives, were from the economically productive age groups of 18–60 years, with the mean age being 35.19 years (Table 2.4ii) and with almost 79 per cent of these losing income due to the absence from work due to caregiving (Table 2.4iii).

The average income lost by employed CGs who lost income due to caregiving was ₹2,695/- for all (₹2,788 if we exclude the single CG whose income loss details were unavailable);[18] with the maximum amount lost being ₹15,000 during the year (Table 2.4ii). Incidentally, an ILO (2003) study which documented the impact on women who took responsibility of ill members, found 44 per cent respondents reporting loss of income ranging from ₹100 to 18,000, with the average loss being ₹2,200 (in Medhini et al. 2007b: 1091). According to Pradhan et al. (2006: xxii), the income lost due to the absence from work of CGs was around 3.5 per cent of the current income of affected HHs. With regard to the present study, the figure pertaining to income lost during the year by those HHs where CGs lost income,[19] taken as a percentage of the total annual HH wage income, was about 5.55 per cent.[20] Among CGs currently not employed, six were employed earlier, with four giving up their job because of caregiving (Table 2.4iv); the earnings of these ranged from ₹600 to 1,560/- per month, with the mean earnings (thus income lost) being ₹1,220 (Table 2.4v).

From all of the above it can be seen that, despite the non-availability of full-time CGs in most cases and that caregiving was done primarily part-time and only when absolutely needed, there has been loss of income due to caregiving in HIV/AIDS HHs, over

Table 2.4iv

Details of CGs currently not employed

	Frequency	% in terms of total HHs	% of HHs in terms of CGs currently not employed
Was CG who is presently not employed, employed earlier			
Yes	6	3	25
No	15	7.5	62.5
Not applicable (students)	3	1.5	12.5
Total	**24**	**12**	**100**
If CG was employed earlier did he or she have to give up employment due to caregiving			
Yes	4	2	66.7
No	2	1	33.3
Total	**6**	**3**	**100**

Source: Author's field work.

Table 2.4v

Amount lost per month by CGs who were working earlier

Minimum (₹)	Maximum (₹)	Mean (₹)	SD
600	1,560	1,220*	537.77

Source: Author's field work.
Note: *This figure is only considering the earnings lost of three individuals since details of the fourth are not available.

and above the regular loss of income on account of death of AIDS earning members and/or loss of income/employment of HIV+ members (see Appendix II: Table AII.ii for summarized details).

Needless to say, caregiving is an area that needs much attention, especially since it involves women, those from the working age-groups, those above 60 years[21] and minors. According to Help Age,[22] 90 per cent of care takes place at home, usually involving older women; according to Medhini et al. (2007b: 1090), the increasing population being left to deal with the burden of care is a major livelihood concern. While having minors/children as CGs can contribute to mental ill health, poor psychosocial development (D'Cruz 2004: 54; Dixit 2005: 110; Medhini et al. 2007a: 563–564) and insufficient education, thereby making them less qualified for more remunerative jobs in the future; women can be a subject of *time poverty*, wherein, besides depletion of financial resources to meet the mounting medical expenses, they face emotional exhaustion, fatigue and burn-out, with the role as CGs being taxing in terms of time and physical exertion (Pradhan and Sundar 2006: 23). Things get accentuated in case of women since they perform not only routine HH tasks, but also caregiving duties and remunerative work, which occasionally includes additional job taken to supplement fast reducing HH income (Medhini et al. 2007b: 1091; UNDP 2003, in Pradhan and Sundar 2006: 23). Additionally, there is an *empowerment cost* when women's time is taken away from other productive work to unpaid care of ill members; it is an opportunity cost which women have to pay since their ability to participate in income generating activities, skill building and leisure activities are reduced drastically (UNAIDS Task Team on Gender and HIV and AIDS, in Pradhan and Sundar 2006: 23).

2.5 Additional Burden: Death of Non-HIV Earning Members

In the sample of HIV/AIDS HHs there were five cases of death of non-HIV infected earning members during the last two years, including that of a member aged 60 years and of another aged

65 years. Pertaining to the study, we can say that 2.5 per cent of the HIV/AIDS HHs witnessed death of at least one HIV-negative member. As opposed to this, there were four instances of death of earning members in non-HIV/AIDS HHs. Incidentally, among the five HIV/AIDS HHs where death was witnessed, in three HHs, an AIDS earning member had also died. These HHs thus bore twice the burden of hardship on account of loss of employment/income (average income lost was about ₹5,250 per month per HH). No HH got compensation from the employers of the dead members.

Table 2.5i provides details pertaining to death of earning non-HIV members; with relative average earnings being lower in HIV/AIDS HHs. Among other reasons, this was primarily due to the fact that in the former, non-HIV members had to often take care of HIV+ members; absenteeism from work thus denied them from earning better incomes. All the dead earning non-HIV members from HIV/AIDS HHs were from lower monthly income brackets, unlike the members from the non-HIV/AIDS HHs who belonged to relatively superior brackets (Table 2.5ii). With regard to the number of months the dead non-HIV members suffered or were

Table 2.5i

Details of dead non-HIV earning members of the last two years

	HIV/AIDS HHs (N = 5)				Non-HIV/AIDS HHs (N = 4)			
	Min.	Max.	Mean	SD	Min.	Max.	Mean	SD
Age (years)	24	65	47.8	16.02	19	50	36	16.35
Earnings of the person per month (₹)	1,500	7,000	3,100	2274.86	2,000	8,000	4,500	2516.61
Number of months suffering/ill	1	24	9.8	9.09	1	12	6.5	6.35
Total amount of money spent on funeral (₹)	1*	10,000	4,340#	4101.93	3,000	20,000	9,500	7593.86

Source: Author's field work.
Notes: *Amount to indicate unknown funeral expenses (expenses were sponsored by somebody outside the household).
If we exclude the unknown funeral expenses of one dead person, mean funeral expenses will be ₹5,425.

Table 2.5ii

Distribution of dead non-HIV earning members based on monthly income slabs

Monthly income slabs	HIV/AIDS HHs			Non-HIV/AIDS HHs		
	No.	Per cent figures for total sample	Per cent figures for only those dead	No.	Per cent figures for total sample	Per cent figures for only those dead
₹1001–2000	2	1	40	1	.5	25
₹2001–3500	2	1	40	0	0	0
₹3501–5000	0	0	0	2	1	50
₹5001–7500	1	.5	20	0	0	0
₹7501–10,000	0	0	0	1	.5	25
Sub-total	*5*	*2.5*	*100*	*4*	*2*	*100*
HHs without non-HIV death	195	97.5		196	98	
Total	**200**	**100**		**200**	**100**	

Source: Author's field work.

ill before dying, the figures were lower for non-HIV/AIDS HHs at 6.5 months as against 9.8 for HIV/AIDS HHs. Field observations revealed that in HIV/AIDS HHs, despite illness, non-HIV members have to often work for longer periods to sustain HH incomes; besides not getting sufficient medical attention due to HIV caused scarcity of HH resources. While in HIV/AIDS HHs even those above 60 years were engaged in earning activities to supplement income, which was not the case in non-HIV/AIDS HHs; amount of money spent on funerals was comparatively close to 50 per cent less in the former (Table 2.5i).

Though the number of deaths pertaining to employed non-HIV members is more or less the same in both samples, the two nevertheless differ substantially on other parameters, with HIV/AIDS HHs standing at a greater disadvantage. Even with regard to the number of deaths of non-HIV employed members, where HIV/AIDS HHs had only one extra death compared to the control group, though the difference appears marginal and inconsequential, it cannot be ruled out, as affirmed by field interactions, that extra death of non-HIV members' take place in HIV/AIDS HHs either because attention with regard to health care is on HIV+ member(s), with non-HIV members not getting sufficient amount since their ailment is not considered 'as serious as HIV/AIDS'; or on account of scarcity of resources caused by high expenses and fall in incomes contributed by HIV/AIDS.

2.6 Other Findings

2.6.1 Coping Mechanisms Pertaining to Income and Employment

HIV/AIDS HHs adopt numerous ways, or coping mechanisms, to address their precarious situation of rising expenses and falling incomes; among these four directly associated with income and employment, as revealed by the study, were: (i) wife of HH head or female HIV+ respondent takes up employment; (ii) minor children take up employment; (iii) those above 60 years take up employment; and (iv) the HIV+ respondent takes an additional job. In the context of the present study, while in 22 per cent HHs the wife/HIV+ female respondent took up employment for the first time; in 5 per cent of the cases those above 60 years of age took employment (Table 2.6.1i). Likewise, while in 6 per cent of the sample HHs the HIV+ respondents took an additional job to sustain dwindling HH income; in 6.5 per cent HHs minor children took up earning activity, with there being cases where the minor children themselves were HIV+. The total number of HIV/AIDS HHs from the study sample adopting the mentioned coping mechanisms, either singly or in combination, was 65 (32.5 per cent).

That the wife/woman has to take up employment is a common occurrence in HIV/AIDS HHs, irrespective of whether it is male-headed or female-headed. In male-headed HHs, the wife often takes up a job due to unemployment or 'un-employability' of the husband, or due to the need of extra income to take care of rising expenses on account of HIV/AIDS. Occasionally, the wife takes

Table 2.6.1i

Coping mechanisms related to income and employment made use of in HIV/AIDS HHs

	No. of HHs based on sex of the HH head			Per cent of total HHs
	Male	*Female*	*Total*	
Wife/HIV+ female respondent takes up job to support HH	24	20	44	22
Children take up job to support HH	2	11	13	6.5
Those above 60 years take up job	7	3	10	5
HIV+ respondent takes up additional job (case of ≥2 jobs)	8	4	12	6

Source: Author's field work.

up employment to compensate for the drop in HH income due to absenteeism of her spouse due to HIV/AIDS. In female-headed HHs, a woman takes up a job on account of death of her spouse, which quite often is due to AIDS itself. With regard to children (those equal to or less than 16 years of age) taking up paid activity to supplement HH income, it is a happening especially witnessed in female-headed HHs, where the woman, usually the mother, is unable to support the HH with her meagre income.[23] Also, children have to work more in female-headed HHs because the female-head herself is often HIV+ and unable to work, or work much. Studies like Pradhan et al. (2006: 43) confirm the higher work force participation rate (WFPR) among children and the elderly in HIV/AIDS HHs as compared to non-HIV/AIDS HHs, wherein it is the female members of the former that are more vulnerable than their male counterparts. The coping mechanisms mentioned are not usual happenings in HHs in general; that they are peculiar to HIV/AIDS HHs can be seen by the fact that all were absent in the control group.

With regard to the issue of working minor children, leaving aside caregiving duties which some do almost single-handedly, the WFPR of children in HIV/AIDS HHs though appearing a small figure, was nevertheless a positive figure, unlike non-HIV/AIDS HHs where it was nil. Dixit (2005: 110) also highlights that demand for children's labour for domestic or income-generating work besides caregiving increases with HIV/AIDS in the HH. Though NCAER/NACO/UNDP findings pertaining to the WFPR among minor children were quite similar to the present study, the two nevertheless differ with regard to the gender of the HIV+ minor working children; while the latter found among the minor employed children, HIV+ males (besides HIV+ females), the former found WFPR only among HIV+ minor females (Pradhan et al. 2006: xxi).

On a related issue pertaining to children, the present study found that 21 (10.5 per cent) HIV/AIDS HHs, of which 17 (81 per cent) were female-headed, withdrew their children aged 16 years and below from educational institutions on account of reasons like 'un-affordability', taking care of HIV+ members, and taking up of remunerative activity. The corresponding figure was nil for non-HIV/AIDS HHs. To compare with the findings of the present study, in Thailand it was found that once a HH member developed AIDS, 15 per cent HHs withdrew their children from school/education (Pitayanon et al. 1997; UNAIDS 2002; Whiteside 2002, in Nielsen and Melgaard 2004: 45). With regard to the present study, though there were more working children in female-headed sample HHs, if one considers the 65 HHs where at least one of the mentioned coping mechanisms was adopted, statistical analysis shows *absence of significant* association between coping mechanisms used and gender of the HH head.

It is but obvious that poorer the HH more would be the need for adoption of coping mechanisms for the sustenance of HHs. The present study effectively found that coping mechanisms were adopted primarily by HHs from the lower income brackets, with statistical tests showing *significant* association between coping mechanisms used and total annual HH income slabs. The coping mechanisms which were totally absent in non-HIV/AIDS HHs, were conspicuous by their absence in case of the relatively better HIV/AIDS HHs as well, barring a couple of exceptions, where the wives had to take up jobs of their spouses who incidentally had their own private businesses (see Appendix II: Table AII.iii).

2.6.2 Loss of Employment/Income for HIV+ Members or CGs during the Last One Year

In 43 (21.5 per cent) HHs there were job losses witnessed during the year as a direct result of HIV/AIDS (Table 2.6.2i). Of the remaining 157 HHs where permanent job loss had not occurred, the status of 24 (12 per cent) HHs was uncertain with regard to future employment, since these had respondents who were currently sick for the last three months or more; though these hoped to resume work post-recovery, their physical state in reality would probably not permit them to do so. Presently 66.5 per cent of the sample HHs had no job loss during the year (though some lost/quit their jobs *over* 12 months earlier). Statistical tests showed *absence of significant* association between gender of the HH head and whether lost job during the year; loss of job was gender independent.

If one considers those HHs where there was loss of income to a HIV+ member or CG during the year on account of HIV/AIDS, the average income lost was ₹15,460 per HH; with the figure becoming ₹3,324 if we consider *all* sample HHs taken together (Table 2.6.2ii). While the amount of money lost during the year was as high as ₹81,000, the income lost per month was as high as ₹9,000. The average time span since members lost their jobs was 5.84 months. Close to 49 per cent of those who lost employment during the course of the last one year lost between

Table 2.6.2i

Details of HIV+ members or CGs who lost job/income during the last one year

	No. of HHs	% of HHs
Lost job	43	21.5
Did not lose job (includes HHs with non-working members)	133	66.5
Presently not working due to illness but hopes to work in the future	24	12
Total	**200**	**100**

Source: Author's field work.

Table 2.6.2ii

Income lost and months not working@

	No. of cases	Min.	Max.	Mean	SD
Total amount actually lost last year (₹)	43	1,000	81,000	15,460#^	15979.70
Income lost per month (₹)	43	500	9,000	2,627*	1796.76
Months without work in last one year	43	1	11	5.84	3.26

Source: Author's field work.
Notes: @Pertaining to HIV+ members or CGs who lost income/employment due to HIV/AIDS during the last one year.
#Mean income lost during the year by all 200 sample HHs was ₹3,324.
^This figure cannot provide per month data since the number of months where HHs lost income last year vary between HHs.
*This figure is useful for arriving at potential loss of income for the following year.

₹5,000 and 15,000, with almost 21 per cent losing in the range of ₹15,001–25,000 and another 14 per cent approximately losing above ₹25,000 (Table 2.6.2iii).

Most of the unemployment which took place during the last 12 months due to HIV/AIDS was in HHs with low total annual

Table 2.6.2iii

Total income lost last year due to loss of job on account of HIV/AIDS

Total income lost	No. of HHs	Per cent in terms of total HHs	Per cent of HHs where loss of job took place
Below ₹5,000	7	3.5	16.3
₹5,000–15,000	21	10.5	48.8
₹15,001–25,000	9	4.5	20.9
₹25,001–50,000	4	2	9.3
₹50,001–75,000	1	.5	2.3
₹75,001–1,00,000	1	.5	2.3
Sub-total	*43*	*21.5*	*100*
Those who did not lose employment	157	78.5	
Total	**200**	**100**	

Source: Author's field work.

incomes (Table 2.6.2iv). Incidentally, the loss of employment itself contributed to HHs to have less income. While lower middle-income HHs become poor, poor HHs become even poorer. The reservoirs of disease among poor populations inevitably prevent HHs from climbing out of poverty-traps (ADB 2004: 3). While the poor are not necessarily more likely to become infected with HIV, the impact of HIV is often magnified in conditions of poverty (see UNAIDS 2008: 162). ADB/UNAIDS (2004) in the same earlier source, reveals that while the financial burden associated with HIV for the poorest HHs in India represents 82 per cent of annual

Table 2.6.2iv

Total income lost last year vis-à-vis total annual HH income of concerned HHs

		Total amount lost last year due to loss of employment on account of HIV/AIDS						
		Below ₹5,000	₹5,000– 15,000	₹15,001– 25,000	₹25,001– 50,000	₹50,001– 75,000	₹75,001– 1,00,000	*Total*
	Up to ₹25,000	1	8	2	0	0	0	**11**
	₹25,001– 50,000	5	7	4	2	1	0	**19**
	₹50,001– 1,00,000	1	4	1	1	0	1	**8**
Total annual HH income slabs	₹1,00,001– 1,50,000	0	2	0	0	0	0	**2**
	₹1,50,001– 2,00,000	0	0	2	1	0	0	**3**
	₹2,00,001– 2,50,000	0	0	0	0	0	0	**0**
	₹2,50,001– 3,00,000	0	0	0	0	0	0	**0**
	₹3,00,001– 5,00,000	0	0	0	0	0	0	**0**
	Above ₹5,00,000	0	0	0	0	0	0	**0**
	Total	7	21	9	4	1	1	**43**

Source: Author's field work.

income, the comparable burden for the wealthiest families was a little over 20 per cent.

As per the findings of the present study, the total income lost during the year was up to ₹15,000 per HH in the case of 28 (65.12 per cent) HHs which lost income, with the percentage going to a whopping high of about 86 per cent if we include those which lost income of up to ₹25,000. In short, while most of the HHs which lost income last year came from lower annual income brackets, the amount lost was less than or equal to ₹25,000 in close to 86 per cent of the cases. To understand in the right perspective the gravity of the situation of what the loss means to HHs, let us assume that the loss of income was ₹15,000 (that is, the approximate mean income lost as shown in Table 2.6.2ii). This loss was greater than 28.5 per cent of the current average annual HH income of the 43 HHs which lost income due to unemployment caused by HIV/AIDS[24] and over 30 per cent of current average HH wage income.[25] Additionally, if we consider that of the 43 HHs losing income during the year, 30 had their current annual HH incomes less than or equal to ₹50,000, the average income lost (@ ₹15,000) represents almost 50 per cent of the total annual HH income,[26] with the current average HH wage income lost being over 56 per cent per HH.[27]

2.6.3 Loss of Double Employment and Sources of Income

As already seen, HIV/AIDS is notorious on its impact on income/employment; it causes death of earning members, leads to absenteeism, inability to work full-time and 'un-employability' due to which HH incomes plummet. CGs losing income/employment is an added concern. The economic impact gets compounded for HHs losing two or more sources of income.

Tables 2.6.3i and 2.6.3ii highlight how 16 (8 per cent) HHs had stronger economic crises than the others on account of experiencing double loss of income during the year. The figure becomes 19 (9.5 per cent) if we add HHs where two earning members died,

Table 2.6.3i

Details of those losing two income sources^*

Total annual HH income	Male-headed HHs	Female-headed HHs	Total
Up to ₹25,000	1	4	5
₹25,001 – 50,000	2	7 + {3}	9 + {3}
₹50,001 – 1,00,000	0	2	2
₹1,00,001 – 1,50,000	–	–	–
₹1,50,001 – 2,00,000	–	–	–
₹2,00,001 – 2,50,000	–	–	–
₹2,50,001 – 3,00,000	–	–	–
₹3,00,001 – 5,00,000	–	–	–
Above ₹5,00,000	–	–	–
Total	3	13 + {3}	16 + {3}

Source: Author's field work.
Notes: ^That of dead working HIV/AIDS or non-HIV/AIDS member and a living member who lost employment during the year due to HIV/AIDS.
*Those which have lost two sources of income due to death—earning AIDS person and earning non-HIV/AIDS person—have been put alongside in parenthesis.

including a non-HIV member. From Table 2.6.3i, two observations come to fore: *firstly*, it is the female-headed HHs which are more adversely affected due to loss of income/employment of two earning members;[28] and *secondly*, the loss of two earning members is witnessed in HHs with lower annual incomes.[29] On a per month basis, the average income lost by the 16 HHs from the two sources was approximately ₹5,248 per HH, which on an annual basis becomes a substantial ₹62,970 per HH; an amount which would have placed them in higher income brackets and better living conditions. The income lost per year as shown, is more in terms of estimated loss of potential future income per annum, based on per month earnings lost.[30] If instead of the mentioned method to calculate average amount of earnings lost by HHs having double loss, the average is calculated by considering each category separately, that is, considering the mean earnings lost by all dead earning HIV/AIDS members' HHs taken separately[31] irrespective of whether there was double loss of income or not and

Table 2.6.3ii

Summarized details of HIV/AIDS HHs pertaining to loss of income

No. of HHs (Per cent represents total sample HHs)	Nature/category of HHs	Average HH income lost per month (₹)	Average HH income lost per annum (₹)
16 (8%)	HHs where two formerly earning members do not contribute to HH income on account of: a) death of an earning AIDS member or earning non-HIV/AIDS member, and b) unemployment of an earning member during the year due to HIV/AIDS caused illness.	5,247.50*	62,970*
19 (9.5%)	HHs where two earning members do not contribute anymore to HH income: these include those from above and 3 HHs wherein besides an earning AIDS member who died, another earning non-HIV/AIDS member has also died.	5,215**	62,580**
43 (21.5%)	HHs where a member has lost job and thus source of income directly on account of HIV/AIDS	2,627	31,524
77 (38.5%)	HHs where AIDS members have died	4,673	56,076
68 (34%)	HHs where earning AIDS members have died^	5,292	63,504

Source: Author's field work.

Notes: *These figures are arrived by considering earnings lost of only the concerned HHs with double loss of employment/income. If we take HHs separately, that is, those that lost earnings of dead AIDS members (68 HHs) and those that lost earnings during the year due to job loss caused by HIV/AIDS (43 HHs), the mean figures get higher at ₹7,918 p.m. and ₹95,016 p.a. per HH having two sources of income lost.
**Figures arrived at in the same way as done above.
^Those whose earnings are known.

mean earnings lost by all those who lost their job during the last 12 months due to HIV/AIDS contributed illness taken separately,[32] the average earnings lost by the double income losing HHs' rises to ₹7,918 and ₹95,016 per month and per annum per HH respectively.

To put things in perspective, had it not been for HIV/AIDS contributed illness and the resulting loss of full time employment, HH incomes of at least 68 (34 per cent) HHs would have been higher by an average of about ₹63,500 per annum; 34 per cent of the HHs would thus have been in higher income brackets (Table 2.6.3ii). To understand the severity of the situation of income lost, we need to note that 147 (73.5 per cent) HHs had their last total annual HH income less than or equal to ₹63,500 per HH. For those having double income loss, if the mean income lost is calculated on the basis of average income lost by the concerned HHs as reflected by (*) in Table 2.6.3ii, income lost will be a whopping high of ₹7,918 per month and ₹95,016 per annum per HH. If we exclude the HIV+ respondents who lost their job over one year back and instead we consider only those (including CGs) who lost their job due to HIV/AIDS during the course of the last one year, the mean earnings lost per HH becomes ₹31,524 (Table 2.6.3ii). The total average income lost by PLWHA currently not working in the last one year, was found to be ₹27,421 by NCAER/UNDP/NACO (Pradhan et al. 2006: xxii). The high amount of income loss, (in)directly attributable to HIV/AIDS, was also found by other studies; Booysen et al. (2002) for instance, reported that in South Africa (in)direct income losses of HHs from HIV/AIDS amounted to more than thrice the average monthly income per capita (in Canning et al. 2006a: 14).

2.6.4 Miscellaneous

Among the sample HIV/AIDS HHs there were some facing far serious throes of despair and economic ordeal than others. The crises was accentuated in HHs where: (i) more than one earning AIDS member had died; (ii) two or more earning members including non-HIV members had lost their job during the course of the last 12 months;[33] and (iii) there was not a single member who was employed during the year. Not only these HHs faced the problem of coping with huge expenses, but also with loan repayments, which in many cases were yet to even commence.

HIV/AIDS has adverse bearing not only on present HH income/ employment as the present study findings have shown, but also on premature morbidity and mortality among sick individuals which can lead to a future fall in income/employment. The adverse fallouts faced by HIV/AIDS HHs can only worsen in years to come. To substantiate the same: (i) many of those presently working are gradually becoming more sick/weak; coupled by insufficient medical treatment and nutrition due to 'un-affordability' they will become unemployable themselves, thereby reducing HH incomes further; (ii) many of those who lost employment/income, have lost it during the course of the last one year; in future their contribution to HH income will be nil, though this year it was positive despite having lost the job; and (iii) children doing paid services or even HH chores and caregiving are deprived of sufficient education, which can deprive them of better earnings in the future. Additionally, if we consider the possibility of the need for future caregiving when present HIV+ members need the same, there will be further drop in HH income.

Losing income/employment due to HIV/AIDS is a serious cause for concern not only because of fall in HH incomes especially in times of rising expenses, but also on account that for the purpose of covering deficits, HHs depend disproportionately on borrowings and 'unrequited and/or unrevealed income' (UUI), the latter which even occasionally includes amounts raised through dubious means (see Glossary and also Pradhan and Sundar 2006: 106). Lost earnings and increased expenses have long-term adverse impacts on HH savings and asset-holdings for a majority of HHs as they are not covered by social security, health and life insurance (see also Ojha and Pradhan 2006: 3). As mentioned earlier as well, members of HIV/AIDS HHs have relatively lower long-term accumulation of human capital in terms of health and education (Ojha and Pradhan 2006: 3). The extent of the long-term adverse economic impact varies according to the initial economic status of the HH, with richer HHs having greater resilience in absorbing the adverse economic shock of AIDS than poorer ones (Basu et al. 1997, in Ojha and Pradhan 2006: 3). Findings of the present study correspond with existing evidence indicating that while individuals/HHs are economically affected by HIV/AIDS, it is the poor and marginalized HHs that are more vulnerable to the impacts than economically well-off ones (see also Bertozzi et al. 2001; Kadiyala and Barnett 2004: 1891). The poor thus get poorer, with the risk of becoming irreversibly impoverished (Medhini et al. 2007b: 1088).

Notes

1. Considered only if it is superior to that of the HH head.
2. HH head was either with an inferior job, was unemployed, retired/housewife or was unable to work due to illness.
3. Contributed by reasons such as 'un-affordability' to pay fees or other expenses related to education; caregiving duties for children; and employment of children for supplementing HH incomes.
4. In developing countries with majority of HIV-infected people being in the age group of 15–45 years, having families and thus dependants, is not uncommon.
5. In 69 per cent of the sample HIV/AIDS HHs, members lived alone as nuclear families, many of who had to do so ever since HIV detection, which forced people to move and stay separately.
6. Though interest is a component of non-wage income the present study only shows if there were interest earnings during the year. Besides numerous constraints (financial, time and manpower) which acted as impediments, the study did not go into details of actual amounts of interest earned due to the following: (i) it is not easy to find correct interest amounts earned by a HH considering various types of savings, savings of different members, savings in different places and savings of different tenures; (ii) HHs usually do not reveal correct interest earnings either because of ignorance or because it reveals the HH savings/investments structure; (iii) actual interest amount earned did not matter significantly for the objectives of the present study since the basic focus was on the last one year HH income and expenditure; to see if the annual income (excluding interest, since it is primarily on past earnings/savings) would suffice to meet the annual expenditure.
7. Presence of more female-headed HIV/AIDS HHs can also be found in other studies like Dixit (2005: 142).
8. Hosegood et al. (2004) indicate that dissolution was four times greater than non-HIV affected HHs (see Avert 2008).
9. http://dsacs.delhigovt.nic.in/naco_policy.asp
10. The impact of HIV/AIDS on income/employment affects adversely not only individuals/HHs, but also economic growth. For illustrative purpose, some channels, (in)directly pertaining to income/employment, through which AIDS affects economic growth include: (i) decline in total factor productivity resulting from increased mortality and morbidity associated with AIDS, (ii) change in skill composition of the labour force due to unequal incidence of AIDS among different grades of labour and (iii) decline in growth rate of the economically

active population because of death caused by AIDS to young adults (Ojha and Pradhan 2006: xiv–xv).

11. Field interactions revealed HIV/AIDS reducing individuals/HHs from 'riches to rags'; and occasionally even from being big time donors/lenders to borrowers, especially post-death of earning male HH heads. The rapid transition from relative wealth to relative poverty on account of HIV/AIDS can be found also in Gaigbe-Togbe and Weinberger (2003: 30) in the context of Zambia.

12. For the purpose of this section, employment details of only one HH member from the working age group of 18–60 years have been considered; while in case of the HIV/AIDS HHs sample the member is the HIV+ respondent, who may or may not be earning, in case of the control group, the member is a presently earning member.

13. The 9 per cent who 'never worked' and 3 per cent who 'worked in between' have been clubbed together to constitute the 'never worked' category, since besides not working at the time of HIV detection, they are not working at present as well.

14. These included agricultural labourers, construction/manual workers, skilled/semi-skilled/non-agricultural labourers, drivers, domestic servants and workers in small shops/petty business.

15. Pertains to all HIV+ respondents who either worked earlier, are presently working, or both; the figure excludes the 24 from the 'never worked' category.

16. This was especially a serious problem in HHs where both parents were HIV+ and children were too small to do caregiving duties.

17. As per an ILO (2003: 3) supported study, CGs who looked after PLWHA were mostly spouses (60 per cent), followed by parents (32 per cent), children (6 per cent) and siblings (2 per cent).

18. The mean income lost for *all* sample HHs' was about ₹406.

19. Taking into consideration the 29 cases whose lost earnings are known.

20. Mean annual HH wage income for the concerned HHs was ₹50,276 (SD. 43355).

21. In some African countries 50–60 per cent of the orphaned children live with their grandparents. In the absence of affordable treatment and schooling, older people face increased financial strain in caring for their adult children and orphaned grand children which increases their poverty. In Tamil Nadu, older people caring for orphaned children reported selling property or pledging it with money lenders for interest rates ranging from 36 to 210 per cent (in Medhini et al. 2007b: 1090).

22. http://www.helpage.org/researchandpolicy/HIVAIDS/factsandfigures (accessed September 2008).

23. Women earn less even in present times, especially with regard to manual/unskilled labour in the unorganized sectors.

24. Mean income: ₹52,340 (SD: 43232).

25. Mean income: ₹48,991 (SD: 44118).

26. Mean income: ₹30,020 (SD: 13356).

27. Mean income: ₹26,620 (SD: 13000).

28. Of the HHs losing double earning members, about 84 per cent were female-headed.

29. The loss of double income itself is primarily responsible for placing the HHs in lower income brackets.

30. The mean income lost per month by the 16 HHs was about ₹3,213 per HH on account of an earning AIDS member dying and ₹2,035 per HH due to loss of employment during the course of the last one year.
31. Mean earnings of the 68 members were ₹5,292, excluding the non-working members and the two members whose earning details were unknown.
32. Forty-three in number, their mean earnings were ₹2,627.
33. In one HH, four members, including one HIV+, had lost their jobs in the last one year. The loss of employment with regard to earning non-HIV member(s) is not always a consequence of HIV/AIDS.

3

Inflow and Outflow of Household Income

The impact of AIDS is no less destructive than war itself, and by some measures, far worse (Kofi Annan [UNAIDS 2000a, in Singhal and Rogers 2006: 204]).

The chapter highlights how the HH rupee is used/spent and how/from where it comes. The chapter also throws light on the nature of differences that exist between HIV/AIDS and non-HIV/AIDS HHs, and how the females fare as compared to men. The study aims at arriving at a broad indicative inflow/outflow pattern of the HH rupee; perfect matching has not been attempted since complete information of income/expenditure heads is not always available and since occasional unaccounted deficits/surpluses were ignored. The latter, insignificant on being rare happenings of only a handful of HHs that too involving figures of less than two per cent, have been ignored on the assumption that 'last month' income/expenditure patterns may not always be proportionate to that of the 'last one year'.[1]

3.1 How and Where the Household Rupee Goes

This section covers three broad areas: HH expenditure, remittances and savings/investments.

3.1.1A Household Expenditure

Household expenditure has been sub-divided into three broad categories: (i) expenditure on food; (ii) regular monthly HH consumption expenditure (excluding food); and (iii) other annual HH consumption expenditure.

3.1.1Aa Monthly Expenditure on Food

One important head of expenditure for any HH is food. In South Africa, average monthly per capita food expenditure of HIV/AIDS HHs was 70 to 80 per cent that of other HHs, though no significant difference was found in total monthly expenditures, likely because of rise in health-related expenditures (Medhini et al. 2007b: 1088). In Thailand, a study found that once a family member developed AIDS, more than half the HH reduced food intake (Pitayanon et al. 1997, in Narain 2004: 29). Likewise, in urban areas of Côte d'Ivoire, food consumption went down by 41 per cent per capita (UNAIDS 2000b, in Adeyi et al. 2001: 10).

If one assumes that total HH income (that is, wage and non-wage income) was the only source of meeting expenses, with reference to the present study, food expenses in relation to total HH income were almost 51 per cent in case of HIV/AIDS HHs and only 37 per cent in case of non-HIV/AIDS HHs. Unlike the control group, the major chunk of HIV/AIDS HH income thus goes for meeting food expenses alone, despite as shown later, a big number of 71 per cent sample HIV/AIDS HHs depending partly or fully on others for free food, as opposed to only 5.5 per cent in case of the non-HIV/AIDS HHs. The high food expenses vis-à-vis total HH income could be considered as an indicator of two things: (i) the comparatively lower HH incomes in general prevailing in HIV/AIDS HHs (see Appendix II: Table AI.ii); and (ii) food, though a basic human need, cannot be compromised much upon, especially in the context of HIV/AIDS, where due to the nature of sickness, care and treatment, proper consumption of balanced food is recommended to ensure a longer and healthier life for the PLWHA (Pradhan et al. 2006: 60).[2] With HIV/AIDS HHs spending a greater proportion of total

HH income on food, less HH income remains for savings or to meet non-food expenditures, due to which, as shown in later sub-sections, HHs are often forced to opt for dissavings, borrowings or even UUI. Needless to say, the above, generally does not happen in non-HIV/AIDS HHs.

The fact that food expenses form a greater portion of total HH income in HIV/AIDS HHs as compared to non-HIV/AIDS HHs, does not reflect though that per capita expenditure on food is likewise high in the former. On the contrary, while per capita monthly food expenses were only ₹698 approximately for members belonging to the HIV/AIDS HHs sample, the corresponding figure was relatively better at about ₹741 for the control group members, despite there being more members in the latter. A comparison of per HH food expenses also shows that non-HIV/AIDS HHs spend more than their counterparts. While monthly food expenses were about ₹2,632 per HIV/AIDS HH, the figure was relatively higher at ₹3,314 per non-HIV/AIDS HH. The difference in food expenses in the two samples, wherein in case of HIV/AIDS HHs though proportion of HH income spent on food was higher, the per capita expenses were lower (opposite for the control group), can be related to the elasticity of expenditure on food being generally less than one[3] (Pradhan et al. 2006: 68).

At the outset itself one can consider the mean values cited and the fact that there were six (3 per cent) HIV/AIDS HHs spending nil amount on food during the last month (none in case of non-HIV/AIDS HHs),[4] as indicators of the adverse impact of HIV/AIDS on consumption of food. Statistical tests show the food expenses between the two samples to be *very significantly* different from one another.[5] As referred to earlier, an overwhelming majority of 68 per cent sample HIV/AIDS HHs got their food 'partly sponsored' and hence got their own personal/HH food expenses reduced. 'Partly sponsored' food refers to food, cooked or uncooked, over and above what is purchased at one's own cost and obtained free regularly, for example, getting food items free once a month from NGOs;[6] getting a meal free at the work place (happens particularly in case of house-maids and those working in hotels/restaurants); getting somebody to pay for part of the food expenses during the month;[7] or even getting extra sponsored food over and above what is actually paid for and shown herein. In the absence of this 'partly sponsored' food, the predicament of HIV/AIDS HHs would have been worse than what it already is. As was mentioned earlier, an additional 3 per cent HIV/AIDS HHs got their food 'fully sponsored', with these not in a position to spend even a single rupee on food. In light of the above, that HIV/AIDS has an adverse bearing on food, can be seen with a comparison of figures for non-HIV/AIDS HHs, where, while only 5.5 per cent of the sample HHs got the benefit of 'partly sponsored' food, there were none depending on 'fully sponsored' food. To put things in perspective, while less than one-third of the HIV/AIDS HHs did not depend on external sources for food assistance, the corresponding figure was a huge 94.5 per cent in case of non-HIV/AIDS HHs.

To find whether the 'nature' of the food consumed by the HIV/AIDS HHs (that is, whether it was 'partly sponsored', 'fully sponsored' or purchased entirely at own cost) was gender (in) dependent, a statistical test was done by merging HHs dependent on 'fully sponsored' food with those with 'partly sponsored' food to arrive at two categories of HHs: those with sponsored food and those with food at own cost. Test results showed *very significant* association existing between the 'nature' of food and gender of the HH head, with female-headed HHs being more dependent on sponsored food, unlike their male counterparts (similar results were found for the non-HIV/AIDS HHs sample, though the same was of no major bearing since very few HHs were dependent on sponsored food).

The distribution of sample HHs on the basis of monthly food expense slabs has been provided in Table 3.1.1Aa. The same highlights from another perspective the adverse impact of HIV/ AIDS on food. While 17 per cent of the HIV/AIDS HHs spent up to ₹1,000 during the last one month on food, including six per cent of the total sample which spent only up to ₹500 (this latter category includes the three per cent HHs which got their food requirements fully sponsored), the corresponding figure was only one per cent in case of the non-HIV/AIDS HHs. Majority of the HHs from both the samples spent between ₹1,001 and ₹5,000 per month, with the

Table 3.1.1Aa
Comparative monthly food expenses

Food expense slabs	HIV/AIDS HHs				Non-HIV/AIDS HHs			
	Male-headed	*Female-headed*	*Total no. of HHs*	*Per cent of HHs*	*Male-headed*	*Female-headed*	*Total no. of HHs*	*Per cent of HHs*
Up to ₹500	8	4	12*	6	0	0	0	0
₹501–1,000	9	13	22	11	0	2	2	1
₹1,001–2,500	49	37	86	43	42	24	66	33
₹2,501–3,500	25	12	37	18.5	57	11	68	34
₹3,501–5,000	16	15	31	15.5	41	9	50	25
₹5,001–7,500	6	1	7	3.5	9	2	11	5.5
₹7,501–10,000	3	1	4	2	2	0	2	1
Above ₹10,000	1	0	1	.5	1	0	1	.5
Total	**117**	**83**	**200**	**100**	**152**	**48**	**200**	**100**

Source: Author's field work.
Note: *Includes six HHs which did not spend any amount on food (their food requirements were fully sponsored). Of these, four were male-headed HHs and two female-headed HHs.

figure being as high as 92 per cent in case of non-HIV/AIDS HHs and a relatively lower figure of 77 per cent in case of the HIV/AIDS HHs. Interestingly, while statistical tests found *absence of significant* association as well as differences between gender of the HIV/AIDS HH head and monthly food expenses, in case of non-HIV/AIDS HHs there was a *very significant* association/difference present. That there was no association or difference between gender and monthly food expenses in case of HIV/AIDS HHs was an important finding of the present study; for this was despite female-headed HHs having significantly lower total annual HH income unlike male-headed HHs (as shown in the previous chapter). Absence of gender based association is an indicator of female-headed HHs making up their significantly low annual HH income by substantially and significantly depending on partly/fully sponsored food (and UUI, as shown in Section 3.2.1Bc).

The primary explanations for the difference in relationship between gender of the HH head and monthly food expenses in the two independent samples as stated above are as follows: (i) In case of HIV/AIDS HHs, a large number of HHs got their food partly/fully sponsored which among other options includes getting part of the expenses reimbursed by others external to the HH (additionally, as was highlighted, there was a significant association between gender of the HH head and 'nature' of food); (ii) Though no significant association was found between gender and coping mechanisms used by HIV/AIDS HHs (see previous chapter), a number of HIV/AIDS HHs, including female-headed HHs had adopted different ways of generating additional resources, such as wife/HIV+ female respondent taking up employment for the first time, taking up of an additional job, minor children being put into remunerative employment, etc.—all of which were conspicuous by their absence in non-HIV/AIDS HHs, including female-headed HHs; (iii) There was a significant association between gender of the HIV/AIDS HH head and dependence on UUI in 'favour' of female-headed HHs (see Section 3.2.1Bc); amount raised via UUI contribute towards meeting food expenses. As a consequence of the above, while in HIV/AIDS HHs death to the male-HH head does not cause severe changes to monthly food expense slabs despite female-headed HHs having significantly lower total annual HH income, in case of non-HIV/AIDS HHs, since the said reasons do not play any substantial role,[8] there is a significant association between gender and monthly food expenses to the disadvantage of female-headed HHs.

To put things differently, in a perspective that could not only help in further understanding why gender of the HH head does not have any significant association with monthly food expenses in HIV/AIDS HHs (though it does in non-HIV/AIDS HHs), but also in understanding the nature of relationship between monthly food expenses and total HH income, is the correlation analysis between total HH income and total monthly food expenses. While there is bound to be and indeed with regard to the present study there was a positive correlation between the two in both samples, the correlation was relatively smaller in case of HIV/AIDS HHs, and higher—and thus stronger—in case of non-HIV/AIDS HHs. This is in a way an indicator that in non-HIV/AIDS HHs if the male-head dies, as the HH income goes down, so also does strongly the monthly food expenses, since the female-heads[9] besides not depending on partly/fully sponsored food (and UUI), also generally do not seek employment or additional employment for self or minor children. If, however, there is no death of the male-heads in non-HIV/AIDS HHs, with higher HH incomes there is significantly higher amount spent on food, especially considering the fact that majority of the sample HHs came from lower economic backgrounds. In case of the HIV/AIDS HHs on the other hand, on account of dependence on partly/fully sponsored food, UUI and coping mechanisms, in the eventuality of death to the male-head, the correlation between the two variables though positive is relatively weaker, since consumption though directly affected will not be so as much as in case of non-HIV/AIDS HHs. Similarly, if there is no death of the male-head in HIV/AIDS HHs, under the assumption that HH income will be intact (or possibly even more), though food expenses/consumption will go up, it will not be as strongly as in case of non-HIV/AIDS HHs on account of huge outflows (especially medical expenses) which HIV/AIDS HHs in particular have to contend with.

Majority of the HIV/AIDS sample HHs at 77 per cent admitted to a perceptible drop in HH food consumption ever since detection of HIV. These admitted to compromising on food due to paucity of funds.[10] In one case an HIV+ person strictly advised by doctors to at least eat a packet of *'Tiger'* glucose biscuits available for ₹5 on days when she could not afford regular food, had no money to buy the same on a regular basis. In another case, a person lived with extremely low levels of food intake despite NGOs providing free food items, since the person on account of acute frailty was not in a position to carry the provision-bag from the NGO centre up to her residence. Among other HHs, a mode frequently adopted to reduce/adjust consumption expenses was dropping consumption of milk totally. Individuals, including babies in the age group of 1–36 months, were deprived of (purchased) milk and were instead given black tea, often without sugar.[11] Consumption of other dairy products, fruits, meat, etc. was either absent or at best restricted to rare occasions only in most HIV/AIDS HHs. While a number of HIV/AIDS HHs had members who had already committed suicide due to serious hardships, including those related to food inadequacies; a number of HIV+ sample respondents themselves had failed in their own suicide attempts, with some contemplating future attempts if things did not improve.

That HIV/AIDS causes food-related hardships to a much larger section of affected HHs can be seen from the fact that besides the 77 per cent HHs which admitted drop in food consumption due to financial constraints, of the remaining which claimed no fall, 34.8 per cent (16 HHs) actually depended on 'partly sponsored' food on a regular basis. Incidentally, all those needing nutritional support do not always get the same from NGOs. As numerous interactions revealed, a number of HIV+ individuals facing financial difficulties, were denied the monthly nutritional support on account of having a relatively good CD-4 count.[12] To accentuate the problem vis-à-vis food especially considering testing times was the fact that many HHs were deprived of subsidized food and other items like kerosene available under the state-controlled Price Distribution System (PDS) due to non-possession of ration-cards, though some still tried to avail of some assistance by borrowing ration-cards from others. It is another matter altogether that the assistance availed by those with ration-cards was not sufficient to meet actual HH needs. The financial crises faced by HIV/AIDS HHs, whether with reference to food or other HH needs can also be seen with another example; in Goa, when the government announced in the year 2008 plans for providing ₹1,000 per month to all HIV+ individuals on anti-retroviral treatment (ART), instances were recorded of infected persons trying to consciously compromise on their health with the intention of reducing their CD-4 count[13] to less than 200 so that they would be put on ART which would then qualify them to receive the monthly assistance (Nair 2008a: 1).[14]

As mentioned earlier, food is a basic necessity; and though it is so universally, the consumption of proper food becomes especially very important for HIV+ individuals. In addition to HIV care/treatment, improved dietary intake is essential to regain lost weight after an OI. As nutrition expert Dr. Prisca Nemapare says, 'Proper nutrition is the best frontline drug for AIDS' (Singhal and Rogers 2006: 125 and 156–157). Good nutrition and medical care can increase body strength and delay the onset as well as frequency of OIs; a person who gets two square meals a day along with quality medical care whenever OIs take place, can live for several years even without ART; those on ART having proper nutrition and medical care, can increase their lifespan by 20 years or more (Gautham 2008: 1). Nutritional intervention studies suggest that early improvements in the energy and protein intake of PLWHA can help build their reserves and reduce vulnerability to OIs (ibid.). Nutritional interventions are a must especially for young children, orphans and mothers (Medhini et al. 2007b: 1085). Incidentally, while being sero-positive increases the body's energy needs and diminishes appetite, it also decreases the body's ability to digest and absorb nutrients. Nutritional status can affect both the efficacy of ART treatment and the patient's ability to adhere to the treatment regime (A. Malavia, in HRLN 2008: 153). The present study revealed that all the HIV+ sample respondents were advised on the need for proper nutrition. Nevertheless, despite the medical recommendation, 68 per cent did not spend any extra amount on food due to inadequacy of funds. Fortunately, a number of these got occasional assistance from NGOs. Pertaining to the remaining 32 per cent (which spent on getting additional food due to recommendations), while the minimum amount spent was a paltry ₹40 per month, it was as high as ₹1,500 per month. While the average amount spent additionally on nutrition was ₹460 per month if we consider the 64 HHs which actually spent additional money, it becomes a paltry ₹147 if all sample HHs are considered together.

In fine, HIV/AIDS HHs are to a disadvantage when it comes to food as compared to their non-HIV/AIDS counterparts; with the adverse impact being such that it cannot be left unattended. Leaving aside that HIV/AIDS members should have proper nutritional standards on account of their state and treatment; food insecurity and malnutrition can actually accelerate the spread of HIV itself—it can increase people's exposure to the virus[15] and/or increase the risk of infection following exposure[16] (Sharma 2006: 150–151; see also A. Malavia, in HRLN 2008: 152). It needs to be further added, that even within the HIV/AIDS HHs, it is often the female-headed HHs which bear significantly the greater burden. A study in Zambia showed female-headed HHs being food-insufficient for an average 3.4 months per year (FAO 2004, in UNAIDS 2006: 85). Incidentally, the present study found to the disadvantage of female-headed HHs a *significant* association between gender of the HH head and the two issues mentioned earlier, namely 'whether there was a drop in food consumption since HIV detection due to financial inadequacies' and 'whether extra amount was spent on buying additional food as recommended'.

3.1.1Ab Regular Monthly Household Consumption Expenditure

'Regular monthly HH consumption expenditure', as the term suggests, refers to all expenses incurred on a monthly basis, excluding food. That there is a significant difference between the two samples to the disadvantage of HIV/AIDS HHs is apparent in Tables 3.1.1Abi and 3.1.1Abii. For instance, while 21 (10.5 per cent) HIV/AIDS HHs, including the six (3 per cent) HHs which were totally dependent on others for food, spent nil amount on fuel/water, the corresponding figure was zero in case of the non-HIV/AIDS HHs (Table 3.1.1Abi). Unlike the case of numbers of HHs involved, from the viewpoint of the average amount spent on fuel/water, the figure is comparatively higher for HIV/AIDS HHs, particularly on account of the fuel component due to the regular heating of drinking water as per medical advice given to HIV+ individuals (Table 3.1.1Abii).

Pertaining to entertainment (movies in theatres/VCDs/DVDs, picnics, dramas, etc.), while only 28 (14 per cent) HIV/AIDS HHs spent on the same, the figure was higher at 59 (29.5 per cent) in case of non-HIV/AIDS HHs. Additionally, related to entertainment, the study found that while 66.5 per cent HIV/AIDS HHs revealed a drop in entertainment since detection of HIV, only 14 per cent felt

Table 3.1.1Abi

Regular monthly HH consumption expenditure details of HHs actually incurring the expenses

	HIV/AIDS HHs					Non-HIV/AIDS HHs				
	N	Min (₹)	Max (₹)	Mean (₹)	SD	N	Min (₹)	Max (₹)	Mean (₹)	SD
Fuel/ water	179	30	800	304	150.7	200	30	600	264	130
Electricity#	135##	20	1,000	217	135.8	167	50	500	225	92.2
House rent	88@	150	6,000	1,053	801	60@@	300	2,000	948	344.3
Transport	195	100	5,000	701	631.4	200	50	2,000	563	441.2
Entertain- ment	28	20	2,300	357	477.2	59	50	500	201	106.3
Telephone	139*	20	2,000	331	360.7	153	20	1,500	299	240.1
Cable/ dish TV	53^	50	300	208	64	85	100	350	248	50.6
Toilet articles	194	20	1,000	243	164.2	200	50	1,000	255	141.1
Alcohol	39	30	3,000	651	717.5	70	50	2,000	428	403.6
Bidi/ cigarettes/ paan	42	10	1,200	234	266.7	43	30	400	97	85.4
Total of all heads	196	120	10,790	2,359	1555.7	200	330	5,380	2,116	1072.8

Source: Author's field work.

Notes: @Additionally there were another 10 HHs on rent, who have either not paid the amounts during the last month on account of financial difficulties or have got their rental amounts paid by externals.

@@Additionally there were two others on rental basis but did not pay for the same (they got others to pay).

*Additional seven HHs had a phone but whose expenses were fully reimbursed by others.

^ Additional one HH had a connection but its expenses were fully reimbursed by others.

In rental cases, the amount is usually taken in the rent amount itself; electricity thus gets reflected as nil.

An additional 13 HHs having the benefit of electricity have either defaulted on payments, have illegally tapped power lines or have expenses fully reimbursed by others.

Table 3.1.1Abii

Comparative regular monthly HH consumption expenditure details of all sample HHs

	HIV/AIDS HHs (N = 200)					Non-HIV/AIDS HHs (N = 200)					Significance of the differences between the two samples'
	Min (₹)	Max (₹)	Mean (₹)	SD	Percent of total	Min (₹)	Max (₹)	Mean (₹)	SD	Percent of total	
Fuel/water	.00	800	272	170.4	11.77	30	600	264	130	12.48	not significant
Electricity	.00	1,000	147	151	6.34	.00	500	187	118.6	8.86	very significant
House rent	.00	6,000	463	745	20.06	.00	2000	284	473.9	13.45	very significant#
Transport	.00	5,000	683	633	29.65	50	2000	563	441.2	26.71	quite significant
Entertainment	.00	2,300	50	215.3	2.16	.00	500	59	108.1	2.78	very significant
Telephone	.00	2,000	230	337	9.95	.00	1,500	228	245.3	10.80	not significant
Cable/dish TV	.00	300	55	97.6	2.38	.00	350	105	127.2	4.98	very significant
Toilet articles	.00	1,000	236	167	10.21	50	1,000	255	141.1	12.05	quite significant
Alcohol	.00	3,000	127	406.4	5.49	.00	2,000	150	313.7	7.09	very significant
Bidi/paan/cigarette	.00	1,200	49	154.2	2.12	.00	400	21	56	0.98	not significant
Total of all heads	.00	10,790	2,312	1575.1	100*	330	5,380	2,116	1072.8	100*	not significant

Source: Author's field work.

Notes: *The percentage figures including the total are in approximate terms.

In case of house rent alone mean is significantly higher for HIV/AIDS HHs; in the case of all remaining heads mean is significantly higher for non-HIV/AIDS HHs.

there was no change, with the remaining 19.5 per cent averring that even before contracting HIV they were not into entertainment. Pertaining to the first two categories of the cited responses, there was *absence of significant* association between drop in entertainment and gender of the HH head; the drop was by and large gender independent.

With regard to cable/dish television (TV), while there were 54 (27 per cent) HIV/AIDS HHs having the same, the number was 85 (44.5 per cent) in case of non-HIV/AIDS HHs. On a related issue, 124 (62 per cent) HIV/AIDS HHs had a TV, with the number being 145 (72.5 per cent) for non-HIV/AIDS HHs. Not only are the numbers of TV sets and cable/dish connections less in HIV/AIDS HHs, but also the ratio of cable/dish connections to TV sets better in non-HIV/AIDS HHs at 58.6 per cent compared to 43.5 per cent for HIV/AIDS HHs. Also, while a number of HIV/AIDS HHs had TV sets in non-working condition due to insufficiency of funds for repairs, there were among those having cable connections, a few who got the same through illegal means like tapping and parallel connections or at best for a mutually settled price (settlement with cable connection owning neighbours and not with cable service providers) as nominal as ₹50 per month, that too not paid on a regular basis. Non-functioning TVs and illegal connections were as good as absent in non-HIV/AIDS HHs.

Table 3.1.1Abi additionally highlights the presence of more HIV/AIDS HHs in rented premises than non-HIV/AIDS ones. This primarily happens because in the former on detection of HIV, members are often forced to move out and stay separate. In a handful of cases, families had to sell their own houses and move into smaller rented premises for the purpose of generating resources to meet increasing expenses. Incidentally, there were HHs whose future in rented premises itself was uncertain since they did not pay rent and electricity bills for upwards of 5–6 months due to financial troubles and were being regularly reminded of eviction or confiscation of HH assets. More HIV/AIDS HHs in rented premises[17] along with relatively fewer HHs having TVs and dish/cable connections, besides less electrical appliances such as washing machines, PCs, fans, audio sets and refrigerators (see Appendix I: Table AI.vii) contributes to the monthly electricity bills of HHs being on an average lower as compared to that of non-HIV/AIDS HHs.

In the case of usage of other regular items such as telephone, transport and toiletries, the numbers were again lesser in case of HIV/AIDS HHs (Table 3.1.1Abi). Additionally, while there were a number of HIV/AIDS HHs depending on external sources for getting certain expenses fully sponsored/reimbursed, there were none when it came to non-HIV/AIDS HHs.[18] Incidentally, number of HHs having members consuming tobacco products was more or less the same in both samples, notwithstanding that average amount spent was different due to the presence of an extreme sample element. In case of alcohol mean amount spent, barring a few exceptions,[19] was generally lower in the HIV/AIDS HHs sample if one considers all HHs (Table 3.1.1Abii); an outcome of medical recommendations given to PLWHA to abstain from alcohol due to illness/treatment.

If one considers the aggregate of 'regular monthly HH consumption expenditure', average expenses per HIV/AIDS HH and per capita per month were approximately ₹2,312 and ₹613 respectively (Table 3.1.1Abii). Surprising that it may sound, these figures were higher than those for the control group where the corresponding figures were about ₹2,116 and ₹473. It needs to be noted that in terms of per capita figures, leaving aside that non-HIV/AIDS HHs were having relatively more members than HIV/AIDS HHs (895 to 754), higher amounts spent by the latter was not an indicator of well being. Amounts were higher in HIV/AIDS HHs primarily due to the higher house rent component,[20] higher amount of travelling expenditure and not to discount, the role played by a couple of extreme sample elements. Similar to the present findings, Pradhan et al. (2006: 60) also revealed that HIV HHs spent a higher proportion of their total consumption expenditure on rent, suggestive of the fact that these HHs have lower assets than non-HIV HHs. It needs to be added that the relatively poor state of HIV/AIDS HHs in terms of expenses on various heads[21] can only worsen if we consider that with regard to a number of HHs, the figures of amounts spent were not entirely of the concerned HHs but of others external to the HHs; in the absence of this assistance, figures mentioned would have been lower than that shown.

Table 3.1.1Abii among other things additionally highlights significant differences existing between the two total sample HHs pertaining to 'regular monthly HH consumption expenditure'. To reduce the number of expense heads, if we merge the percentage figures of cable/dish TV with entertainment; electricity with fuel/water; and alcohol with tobacco products, the distribution of regular monthly HH expenses highlights among others three differences: (i) in HIV/AIDS HHs, there was a relatively smaller share of total expenditure on entertainment; (ii) the share of house rent was comparatively larger in HIV/AIDS HHs; and (iii) in non-HIV/AIDS HHs, the fuel/water/electricity component was relatively higher.

If for comparative purpose, we include monthly HH food expenditure to the 'regular monthly HH expenditure', the expense distribution will appear as in Figure 3.1.1Ab, wherein the food component forms the largest chunk in both categories of HHs, with the same being higher at 61.04 per cent in non-HIV/AIDS HHs, as compared to 53.23 per cent in HIV/AIDS HHs. That HIV/AIDS HHs spend a relatively lower proportion of their total consumption expenditure on food than non-HIV/AIDS HHs was also found by Pradhan et al. (2006: 59).

If we consider total 'regular monthly HH consumption expenditure' (excluding food) as the only outflow and relate it as percentage of total HH income, the proportion of the same for all HHs becomes 44 per cent in case of the HIV/AIDS HHs sample and 23.6 per cent for the non-HIV/AIDS HHs sample. The difference in proportion arises primarily due to differences in total annual HH income itself and due to the relatively higher rent and monthly travelling expense components in case of the HIV/AIDS HHs.

Travelling expenditure needs a brief overview, especially since it got mentioned earlier. HIV/AIDS HHs face a paradoxical situation vis-à-vis travelling needs. While per HH travelling expenses are relatively higher for HIV/AIDS HHs, the expenses are nevertheless insufficient to meet actual needs, which is generally not the case

Figure 3.1.1Ab

Comparative distribution of regular monthly HH consumption expenditure including food

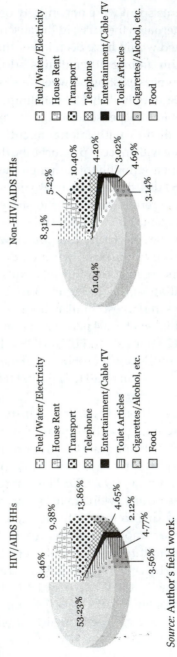

Source: Author's field work.

with non-HIV/AIDS HHs. There is much compromising done by the members of HIV/AIDS HHs, despite part of the travelling expenses being occasionally sponsored/reimbursed by others such as NGOs. To put things in perspective from another point of view, travelling costs are relatively higher in HIV/AIDS HHs despite only 35 per cent HHs having personal two/four wheelers as compared to almost 50 per cent in case of non-HIV/AIDS HHs (see Appendix I: Table AI.vii). The fact of the matter is that HIV+ members regularly need to travel on account of medical reasons, including checkups, ART treatment, CD-4/*viral load* count test, treatment of OIs, etc. Despite the higher average travelling costs and that in a number of cases there is reimbursement of the same, a number of HIV/AIDS HHs face serious financial problems such that besides compromising on medical visits to save on travel expenses, and making even primary-school going children walk long distances each day, with some HHs even contemplating withdrawing children from schools on account of the travelling cost burden, many adult HH members including HIV+ members and senior citizens resort to walking long distances of even 4–5 km on a regular basis, or asking neighbours to do market purchases of goods to reduce paid trips by public transport. Many HHs having native place outside the state, either refrain from visiting the same on account of financial difficulties, or travel in the cheapest 'no reservation'/general class, with some even travelling without proper tickets.

Table 3.1.1Abiii shows a comparative distribution of the two samples on the basis of 'regular monthly HH consumption expenditure' slabs, with the distribution of HHs being positively skewed in nature. Statistical tests found a *significant* association between gender of the HIV/AIDS HH head and 'regular monthly HH consumption expenditure', the same being to the disadvantage of female-headed HHs. Statistical tests also brought to fore *highly significant* differences existing vis-à-vis expenses in relation to gender of the HH head. In case of the non-HIV/AIDS HHs as well, similar differences were found. Death of the male-head obviously has an adverse bearing on 'regular monthly HH consumption expenditure' (excluding food) of both samples.

Table 3.1.1Abiii

Comparative regular monthly HH consumption expense slabs (excluding food)

Expense slabs	HIV/AIDS HHs				Non-HIV/AIDS HHs			
	Male-headed	*Female-headed*	*Total HHs*	*Per cent of HHs*	*Male-headed*	*Female-headed*	*Total HHs*	*Per cent of HHs*
Up to ₹1,000	14	18	32	16	14	12	26	13
₹1,001–2,000	34	33	67	33.5	59	20	79	39.5
₹2,001–3,000	29	20	49	24.5	48	10	58	29
₹3,001–4,000	23	9	32	16	23	5	28	14
₹4,001–5,000	8	1	9	4.5	5	0	5	2.5
Above ₹5,000	9	2	11	5.5	3	1	4	2
Total	**117**	**83**	**200**	**100**	**152**	**48**	**200**	**100**

Source: Author's field work.

3.1.1Ac Other Annual Household Consumption Expenditure

'Other annual HH consumption expenditure' excludes food and regular monthly HH consumption expenditure, except that related to travelling. From the point of view of numbers of HHs involved, that a relatively higher number of HIV/AIDS HHs are at a comparative disadvantage pertaining to various heads can be seen from Table 3.1.1Aci. It needs to be noted that HH figures pertain to only those which have actually spent own money, though part of it may have been later reimbursed by others, or though they may have got additional benefits through external assistance as well. As was with 'regular monthly HH consumption expenditure', here also HHs which got benefits fully sponsored, have been excluded.

Among the various fallouts of HIV/AIDS on HHs, while one is reduced non-health consumption expenditure (Bechu 1998; Booysen et al. 2002), another is reduced nutrition and children's education (Booysen et al. 2002; Donovan et al. 2003, Nampanya-Serpell 2000, all in Canning et al. 2006a: 3). As can be seen from Table 3.1.1Aci with regard to numbers of HHs involved, HIV/AIDS HHs are a disadvantage with regard to all listed heads barring one (that too

Table 3.1.1Aci

Comparative 'other annual HH consumption expenditure' details for concerned HHs

	HIV/AIDS HHs					Non-HIV/AIDS HHs				
	N	Min (₹)	Max (₹)	Mean (₹)	SD	N	Min (₹)	Max (₹)	Mean (₹)	SD
Clothing/footwear	169	50	5,0000	3,147	4627	200	200	25,000	2,693	2726
Automobile	10	4,500	86,000	32,950	28500	6	2,000	3,00,000	73,667	112777
Electronic/electrical appl.	26	650	72,000	6,656	14176	30	300	17,000	3,887	4475
Other durable goods	14	50	5,500	2,193	1998	81	200	10,000	1,643	2009
Education of children	107#	300	1,50,000	6,014	16883	144	100	1,00,000	4,722	10149
Medical (OPD, reg. monthly treat., cost of medicines, etc.)	183□	200	5,00,000	14,197	39909	139	10	26,000	3,676	5577
Travel	196^	500	60,000	8,699	7674	200	800	25,000	7,238	5284
Repair/taxes/insurance/maint. of house/vehicle, etc.	94*	60	1,50,000	5,857	17203	145	50	1,50,000	3,528	14202
Other exp.(wedding/parties/feasts, etc.)	57@	300	4,00,000	13,137	53807	129	200	4,00,000	8,386	37796
Total other annual HH consumption exp. (as per above heads)	196	1,200	5,47,000	37,280	63920	200	1,000	4,55,000	27,311	45038

Source: Author's field work.

Notes: #The actual number of HHs with children of school going age was 128. Of these, while 15 were fully dependent on others for assistance, six withdrew children from school during the year.

□ Another nine HHs had medical expenses but the same were fully reimbursed/sponsored by others.

*An additional three HHs had major expenses but they have not been considered herein since they were fully sponsored by externals.

^An additional four HHs which spent nil amount of their own and got their expenses fully paid by others have been excluded.

@An additional HH had major expenses but the same have been excluded since the same was fully paid by others.

inconsequential considering the few number of HHs involved) related to purchase of automobiles. On a comparative basis, there were fewer HIV/AIDS HHs spending on clothing/footwear, electronic/electrical appliances, other durable goods (furniture, utensils, etc.), education of children, travel, repair/maintenance of house/vehicle, etc.; besides those incurring expenses on weddings, ceremonies and functions. Other than automobiles, the only item where there were more HIV/AIDS HHs was that pertaining to medical expenses.

AIDS threatens the educational system and undermines the social capital of the country (UNAIDS 2000b, in Adeyi et al. 2001: 10). As UNAIDS (2002) reports, in Swaziland and the Central African Republic, school enrolment fell by 25–30 per cent due to AIDS (in Avert 2008). With regard to education in the present study, there were 128 HIV/AIDS HHs with children of school going age (144 non-HIV/AIDS HHs) of which only 107 actually spent of their own income on education (many of these additionally depended for education related assistance on others such as NGOs). Of the rest, while 15 HHs were fully dependent on others for assistance, six HHs withdrew children from school during the last one year on account of financial reasons, including 'un-affordability' of school uniforms and tuition fees and/or the need to perform remunerative or caregiving duties.

Pertaining to the issue of withdrawing children from school, if we consider the time period ever since HIV detection, there were 21 (10.5 per cent) HIV/AIDS sample HHs which withdrew at least one child below the age of 16 years from school due to aforementioned reasons. Unlike HIV/AIDS HHs, there was none of a similar nature in the control group. Besides adverse bearing of insufficient education on the long-term macroeconomic development, children not getting sufficiently qualified could also reflect in their inability to get better jobs in the future. Incidentally, with low salaries, the children's children could as a consequence also end up with less human capital; with the adverse effects of HIV/AIDS thus persisting through generations (Sharma 2006: 120). Pradhan et al. (2006: 60) reiterate that the long-term impact could be more acute, especially if the children are orphaned. Incidentally, because of lack of education, many of those at a higher risk of HIV infection are unable to comprehend the risks and benefits, with up to 90 per cent of those infected daily not knowing about it for almost a decade (Drummond and Kelly 2006: 3).

Interestingly and paradoxically, while with regard to numbers of HHs the HIV/AIDS sample was at a comparative disadvantage, with regard to average amount spent on education the figures were comparatively higher than those of the non-HIV/AIDS HHs sample (Table 3.1.1Aci);[22,23] albeit often assisted through part/full reimbursement by others, dependence on UUI and/or borrowings. In case of education (besides clothing/footwear) though average amount spent by the concerned HHs actually incurring expenditure was higher in the HIV/AIDS HHs sample, with reference to the total sample, the average amount spent was higher in case of the non-HIV/AIDS HHs. Also, in terms of total amount spent on 'other annual HH consumption expenditure', the proportion of expenses of non-HIV/AIDS HHs on education (and clothing/footwear) was higher in case of non-HIV/AIDS HHs (Table 3.1.1Acii). Incidentally, on the issue of education approximately 47 per cent of the HIV/AIDS HHs having children of school going age felt there was a drop in HH expenses vis-à-vis education due to HIV. Statistical tests showed *quite significant* association existing between the perceived drop in education and gender of the HH head, to the disadvantage of female-headed HHs. Seeing that HIV/AIDS does adversely influence education, it appears that the assumption made by studies such as Bell et al. (2003) that one of the channels of impact of HIV/AIDS is through reduced HH expenditure on education, is empirically sustainable (in Pradhan et al. 2006: 62 and 81). Low levels of expenditure on education by HIV/AIDS HHs in general, is reflective not only of lower enrolment levels (ibid.) or possibly higher enrolment in government/aided schools, but also additionally on the assistance received from NGOs. The poor relative position of HIV/AIDS HHs vis-à-vis education can get worse with regard to attainment of higher education in the future.

Other than education, if one looks at Table 3.1.1Aci for numbers of HHs having medical expenses during the last one year, 192 (96 per cent) HIV/AIDS HHs had to bear expenses, of which nine HHs

Table 3.1.1Acii

Comparative 'other annual HH consumption expenditure' details of all sample HHs

	HIV/AIDS HHs (N = 200)				Non-HIV/AIDS HHs (N = 200)					Significance of differences between samples
	Min (₹)	Max (₹)	Mean (₹)	SD	Per cent of total	Min (₹)	Max (₹)	Mean (₹)	SD	Per cent of total	
Clothing/footwear	.00	50,000	2,659	4,402	7.28	200	25,000	2,693	2,726	9.87	significant
Automobile	.00	86,000	1,648	9,411	4.51	.00	3,00,000	2,210	21,870	8.10	not significant
Electrical/electronic appliances	.00	72,000	865	5,503	2.37	.00	17,000	583	2,203	2.14	not significant
Other durable goods	.00	5,500	154	759	0.42	.00	10,000	666	1,509	2.44	very significant
Education	.00	1,50,000	3,218	12,683	8.81	.00	1,00,000	3,400	8,862	12.45	very significant ^
Medical (OPD, treatment, medicines, etc.)	.00	5,00,000	12,991	38,372	35.57	.00	26,000	2,555	4,945	9.36	very significant
Travel	.00	60,000	8,525	7,694	23.26	800	25,000	7,238	5,284	26.56	not significant
Repair/taxes/insurance/maintenance of house/vehicle, etc.	.00	1,50,000	2,667	12,044	7.46	.00	1,50,000	2,558	12,184	9.38	very significant ^^
Other expenses (wedding/parties/religious ceremonies, etc.)	.00	4,00,000	3,744	29,156	10.25	.00	4,00,000	5,409	30,579	19.78	very significant
Total 'other annual HH consumption exp.' (as per above heads)	.00	5,47,000	36,535	63,491	100*	1,000	4,55,000	27,311	45,038	100*	very significant

Source: Author's field work.

Notes: *Percentage figures are in approximate terms only.

^If HHs without children are excluded, differences between the two samples becomes 'quite significant' only.

^^If HHs without 'house repair…' expenses are excluded, difference becomes 'quite significant' only.

got their expenses fully sponsored by others. Only eight (4 per cent) HIV/AIDS HHs were free from medical expenses during the year. Of the 183 (91.5 per cent) HHs which actually bore medical expenses of their own, while a number got part of the same reimbursed by others subsequently, another 14 got additional amounts sponsored by others over and above the actual expenses shown herein. With regard to non-HIV/AIDS HHs, while 61 (30.5 per cent) did not have any medical ailment necessitating expenses, there were nil HHs depending on assistance of others.

In the case of annual expenditure on clothing/footwear, a reference to which was made earlier, while with regard to number of HHs, HIV/AIDS HHs were at a disadvantage with 31 (15.5 per cent) spending nil amount as opposed to none from the control group; with regard to the mean amount spent by the concerned HHs, however, the HIV/AIDS HHs were at an advantage. Notwithstanding the same, the general perception in HIV/AIDS HHs with regard to clothing/footwear was that there was a drop in the same on account of HIV/AIDS, as was indicated by 80.5 per cent HHs. Related to this perception, statistical analysis showed a *very significant* association existing between the same and gender of the HH head, with female-headed HHs experiencing the fall more.

Related to the other heads of expenses like repair/maintenance of house/vehicle, there were instances of HIV/AIDS HHs which did not spend any amount despite urgent need due to financial reasons. There were HHs which had part of their residence in a dilapidated state, with other parts structurally on the verge of collapse due to non-maintenance. Likewise, while only 14 (7 per cent) HIV/AIDS HHs spent money to buy 'other durable goods' during the last one year, in case of the control group there were 81 (40.5 per cent) HHs. Similarly, in case of expenditures on festivities/celebrations, the number of non-HIV/AIDS HHs was higher at 129 (64.5 per cent), as compared to only 57 (28.5 per cent) HIV/AIDS HHs. However, despite the aforesaid fact, it was found that in case of HIV/AIDS HHs there was an occasional tendency in some to splurge, as was witnessed in three HHs during the last one year and another six HHs in the previous year. This tendency, rare but not unknown, happens on account of the mental frame wherein the perception often voiced is, *'contracting HIV/AIDS means all is lost, and hence before one dies it would be better to have a last celebratory get-together, even if one has to borrow or resort to dissavings when all members are alive'.*

Table 3.1.1Acii shows comparative details of all sample HHs taken together. It also highlights expenditure items where there are significant differences between the two samples. Leaving aside mean values pertaining to HH expenses on celebrations and on purchase of 'other durable goods' which were relatively and significantly higher in non-HIV/AIDS HHs, the mean values which were substantially and significantly higher in HIV/AIDS HHs were those pertaining to medical expenses, with the medical expenses of HIV/AIDS HHs being over five times the size as compared to the expenses of non-HIV/AIDS HHs.[24] Incidentally, the increase in HH medical expenditures due to HIV/AIDS is likely to be met by reduction in other expenses. For HHs that are below or close to the poverty line, it can imply reduced expenditure on even essential items such as food and clothing; it can also imply reduced spending on education, which could ultimately contribute in reducing the future stock of human capital (Pradhan et al. 2006: 59).

From Table 3.1.1Acii it can be seen that from the total sample perspective, the percentage expenditure of non-HIV/AIDS HHs on each head (barring medical expenditure and expenditure on electronic/electrical appliances) was higher than their HIV/AIDS counterparts. Incidentally, expenses of the former on electronic/electrical appliances were partly lower because the basic items were already owned by the HHs. From percentage figures point of view, non-HIV/AIDS HHs were relatively better vis-à-vis educational expenses of children and expenses on ceremonies/weddings. HIV/AIDS HHs, on the other hand, besides having an apparently less advantage with regard to purchase of 'other durable goods', had a very high share of medical expenses in relation to total expenses at over one-third the amount at 35.57 per cent, unlike non-HIV/AIDS HHs whose share was only 9.36 per cent. In the case of HIV/AIDS HHs, in terms of size, medical expenses were followed by travel expenses. To show the influence the two bear on total 'other annual HH consumption expenditure', if the same are ignored, 19 (10.5 per cent) HIV/AIDS HHs get their 'other annual HH consumption expenditure' as nil. Unlike HIV/AIDS HHs, in case of the control group, the major expenses in percentage terms were those related to travel. Incidentally, though proportion of the same in the control group was high, comparatively, it was close to the figures of HIV/AIDS HHs. Proportionately, medical expenses formed less than 10 per cent of the total 'other annual HH consumption expenditure' in non-HIV/AIDS HHs.

Table 3.1.1Aciii highlights the positively skewed distribution of HHs with regard to 'other annual HH consumption expenditure'. While in the lower three slabs of up to ₹20,000 there were comparatively more non-HIV/AIDS HHs; from ₹20,001 and upwards expenditure cases, there were relatively more HIV/AIDS HHs barring one exception. Much of the said distribution is caused by the high medical expenses prevalent in HIV/AIDS HHs. Incidentally, while statistical tests have shown *absence of*

Table 3.1.1Aciii

Comparative distribution of HHs based on 'other annual HH consumption expenditure'

Expense slabs	HIV/AIDS HHs				Non-HIV/AIDS HHs			
	Male-headed	Female-headed	Total HHs	Per cent of HHs	Male-headed	Female-headed	Total HHs	Per cent of HHs
Up to ₹5,000	5	9	14	7	9	10	19	9.5
₹5,001–10,000	16	12	28	14	33	13	46	23
₹10,001–20,000	32	21	53	26.5	44	11	55	27.5
₹20,001–30,000	25	18	43	21.5	33	6	39	19.5
₹30,001–50,000	15	15	30	15	13	4	17	8.5
₹50,001–75,000	8	6	14	7	11	2	13	6.5
₹75,001–1,00,000	9	0	9	4.5	4	1	5	2.5
₹1,00,001–2,00,000	2	1	3	1.5	3	1	4	2
Above ₹2,00,000	5	1	6	3	2	0	2	1
Total	117	83	200	100	152	48	200	100

Source: Author's field work.

significant association as well as differences[25] between gender of
the HH head and 'other annual HH consumption expenditure'
for HIV/AIDS HHs; in case of non-HIV/AIDS HHs, however, the
association/differences were found to be *significant*. The findings
are indicators that, while in non-HIV/AIDS HHs on account of
death to the male-head, the female-head experiences reduction
in HH expenses, in HIV/AIDS HHs annual expenditures are
by and large gender independent (despite female-headed HHs
having comparatively lower total annual HH income as seen
earlier). The latter is primarily on account of: (i) adoption of
different coping mechanisms (including dependence on UUI) by
female-headed HIV/AIDS HHs; (ii) the general prevalence of high
medical expenses irrespective of the gender of the HH head; and
(iii) partly due to the assistance received at times in the form of
reimbursements through external sources such as NGOs.

If we consider 'other annual HH consumption expenditure'
as the only expenditure/outflow (excluding food and 'regular
monthly HH consumption expenditure') and relate it to the total
annual HH income, while in case of HIV/AIDS HHs, the proportion
of the same is about 58 per cent, in the case of non-HIV/AIDS HHs,
it is much lower at 25.40 per cent; the main factor contributing to the
difference being the huge medical expenses prevalent in the former.

3.1.1B Remittances

Besides the direct outflow of money on HH consumption, inclusive
of food, regular monthly HH expenditure and other annual HH
expenditure, outflow also takes place via remittances. For the
purpose of this study, remittances include any monetary outflow
in the form of loan repayments, donations, assistance provided to
relations, unilateral payments, etc., wherein at the time of outgoing
there is no *quid pro quo*. In case of HIV/AIDS sample, 43 (21.5 per
cent) HHs indicated that they made remittances in the last one
year; for 33 of these (76.7 per cent of the concerned) remittances
were in the nature of loan repayments. The corresponding
figures for non-HIV/AIDS HHs were 26 (13 per cent); with

Table 3.1.1B

Comparative amount of remittances in the last one year

	HIV/AIDS HHs				Non-HIV/AIDS HHs			
N	Min (₹)	Max (₹)	Mean (₹)	SD	N	Min (₹)	Max (₹)	Mean (₹)	SD
43	250	1,35,000	13,141	24,316	26	300	15,000	5,262	4,708
200	.00	1,35,000	2,825	12,413	200	.00	15,000	684	2,435

Source: Author's field work.

22 (84.6 per cent) HHs making remittances in the form of loan repayments (Table 3.1.1B).

If remittances were the only head of outflow, the ratio of the same to the total annual HH income would be 4.48 per cent for HIV/AIDS HHs and a much lower figure of 0.64 per cent for non-HIV/AIDS HHs. The mean value of remittances of all HIV/AIDS HHs taken together standing at ₹2,825 was 4.13 times higher than that of all non-HIV/AIDS HHs (mean: ₹684). The figure of remittances was lower in the latter HHs since borrowings were relatively lesser. Understandably, statistical tests show the HH remittances of the two samples to be *significantly* different.

3.1.1C Savings and Investments

Among the major economic fallouts of HIV/AIDS, one that has received much attention is the reduction in savings rate (Over 1992; Cuddington 1993; Pradhan et al. 2006). HIV/AIDS broadly contributes to the decline in savings rate on account of: (i) fall in earnings/employment, (ii) increase in medical treatment expenses and (iii) pessimistic expectations of some PLWHA of a shorter lifespan. The shortened expected lifespan while diminishing the incentive to save, can additionally lead to limiting capital accumulation (Arndt and Lewis 2000) and diminishing incentives to invest in education, since the payoff to human capital investments decreases with falling life expectancy (Ferreira and Pessoa 2003, both in Werker et al. 2007: 18).

That HIV/AIDS HHs are to a disadvantage over their relatively matched non-HIV/AIDS counterparts with regard to savings/investments is evident in the present study as well. While only 50 (25 per cent) of the former saved/invested during the last one year, the corresponding figure was as high as 156 (78 per cent) in case of the latter. Details of savings/investments of the sample HHs have been provided in Table 3.1.1Ci. Figures show that whether it is the mean amount of savings per concerned HHs actually saving, mean savings for all sample HHs taken together or even maximum and mean amount saved in different modes, barring the odd case of average amount spent on the purchase of jewellery, the figures for non-HIV/AIDS HHs were superior to those of HIV/AIDS HHs. Incidentally, even in case of jewellery, though mean was less for non-HIV/AIDS HHs, the number of HHs involved in purchases were higher than HIV/AIDS HHs; the figures being 35 to four. While there were comparatively more non-HIV/AIDS HHs at 32 having more than one mode of saving during the year, the figure was only two in case of HIV/AIDS HHs. It is pertinent to add that although during the last one year both sample HHs did not save/invest in the form of purchase of land or house, the position of non-HIV/AIDS HHs was superior to that of HIV/AIDS HHs (see Appendix I: Table AI.vii), wherein 27 and 71.5 per cent of the former owned land/plot and house respectively, with the corresponding figures being only 18.5 and 51 per cent in case of HIV/AIDS HHs; with 2.99 and 2.40 per cent of the latter HHs even selling (earlier) house property and agricultural land respectively on account of HIV/AIDS.

With regard to the issue of HH savings and whether it is gender related, statistical tests showed that while there was *no significant* association between the two in HIV/AIDS HHs, there was a *very significant* association in case of non-HIV/AIDS HHs, to the disadvantage of female-headed HHs. This shows that while savings were adversely affected in female-headed non-HIV/AIDS HHs, apparently due to the death of the male-head, in HIV/AIDS HHs savings were independent of gender of the HH head. Besides the above, statistical tests also highlighted the *absence of significant* differences in savings in HIV/AIDS HHs on the basis of gender,

Table 3.1.1Ci

Comparative savings/investments (including modes of savings) in the last one year

| | HIV/AIDS HHs | | | | | Non-HIV/AIDS HHs | | | | |
	N	Min (₹)	Max (₹)	Mean (₹)	SD	N	Min (₹)	Max (₹)	Mean (₹)	SD
Cash/bank deposits	48	600	2,00,000	25,863	38,983	153	400	2,05,000	27,266	38,951
Purchase of jewellery	4	4,500	49,000	25,375	18,309	35	2,000	2,00,000	20,623	34,113
Purchase of agricultural land	0	–	–	–	–	0	–	–	–	–
Purchase of house/flat	0	–	–	–	–	0	–	–	–	–
Purchase of shares	1	4,000	4,000	4,000	–	1	30,000	30,000	30,000	–
Total Savings (concerned HHs only)	**50**	**600**	**2,00,000**	**26,614**	**41,156**	**156**	**400**	**2,50,000**	**31,561**	**44,009**
Total Savings (all HHs)	**200**	**.00**	**2,00,000**	**6,654**	**23,464**	**200**	**.00**	**2,50,000**	**24,617**	**40,992**

Source: Author's field work.

though there were *very significant* differences present in case of non-HIV/AIDS HHs.

Savings/investments as a proportion of 'total annual HH income',[26] gets to be about 10.56 per cent in case of HIV/AIDS HHs and 22.88 per cent in case of non-HIV/AIDS HHs. However, while in the latter, matching of savings as a proportion to annual HH income does happen to a great extent, in case of the former it does not, since besides savings not being the only head, there is also much of borrowing and UUI. Considering this reality prevalent in HIV/AIDS HHs, the actual proportion of savings to total HH income would be lower than mentioned (see Figure 3.1.2). Savings/investments of the entire control group were almost 3.70 times the size as that of HIV/AIDS HHs sample; or to put differently, savings in the latter were only 0.27 times the size than that in the former. Expectedly statistical tests showed the differences in saving/investment of the two samples to be *very significant* in nature. Comparing the mean values of savings with dissavings for all HHs, while savings were only 0.76 times the size of dissavings in HIV/AIDS HHs indicative of net negative savings, the figure was much higher and superior 5.14 in case of non-HIV/AIDS HHs, an indicator of net positive savings. That unlike the presence of comparatively high savings/investments in non-HIV/AIDS HHs there was large negative savings in HIV/AIDS HHs has been dealt with further in Section 3.2.1Ba.

To look at the saving/investment of HHs from another viewpoint, paradoxically one may say, of those who claimed they saved during the course of the last one year, while a few 'saved' not through employment related earnings but by selling HH items, 14 HIV/AIDS HHs which saved (28 per cent of those saving) alongside also dissaved during the same time. Incidentally, in the case of eight of these 14 HHs, dissavings were greater than savings; in reality these HHs thus had net negative savings. Similarly, if one considers all HHs which had both savings and dissavings, the average savings were less than the average dissavings (in both categories of HHs; see Table 3.1.1Cii). Unlike HIV/AIDS HHs, in the case of non-HIV/AIDS HHs a relatively small figure of only four of the 156 HHs had dissavings along with savings. Among those HHs which saved

Table 3.1.1Cii

Comparative details of HHs which saved and dissaved at the same time

	HIV/AIDS HHs (N = 14)				Non-HIV/AIDS HHs (N = 4)			
	Min (₹)	*Max* (₹)	*Mean* (₹)	*SD*	*Min* (₹)	*Max* (₹)	*Mean* (₹)	*SD*
Total dissavings	2,500	3,00,000	34,964	77,689	2,000	2,75,000	86,000	1,29,453
Total savings	600	1,00,000	19,693	28,539	2,000	2,00,000	63,500	93,771

Source: Author's field work.

and dissaved during the year, while the minimum and maximum figures pertaining to dissavings were higher in HIV/AIDS HHs, it was the non-HIV/AIDS HHs which had the better figures in terms of savings (Table 3.1.1Cii). Incidentally, unlike earlier cited trends, mean dissavings were relatively higher in non-HIV/AIDS HHs. If we, however, consider that average savings in non-HIV/AIDS HHs were comparatively bigger, the ratio between savings and dissavings is relatively superior for non-HIV/AIDS HHs, where savings were 0.74 of the size of dissavings; whereas, it was only 0.56 in case of HIV/AIDS HHs.

3.1.2 Total Outflow

Figure 3.1.2 shows the total outflow of income, that is, how the HH rupee is spent or used annually. The figure is obtained through summation of figures mentioned earlier. For the purpose of getting a proper perspective, a few heads have been redone herein; while regular monthly non-food consumption expenditure excludes travelling expenses, 'other annual HH consumption expenditure' excludes medical and travelling expenses, since the same have been highlighted separately on account of their major role in the total annual outflow.

As highlighted in Figure 3.1.2, the primary differences in the way the HH rupee is used in the two samples are: (i) medical expenses are higher at 13.38 per cent in case of HIV/AIDS HHs

Figure 3.1.2

Where and how the HH rupee goes during the year

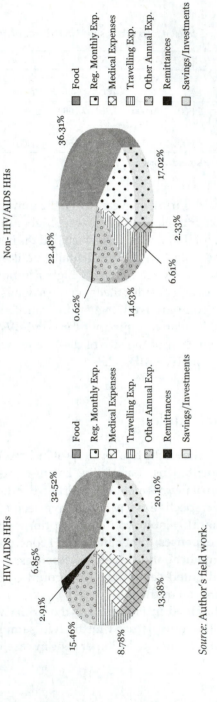

Source: Author's field work.

as compared to only 2.33 per cent for non-HIV/AIDS HHs;[27] (ii) savings/investments were only 6.85 per cent in HIV/AIDS HHs as compared to 22.48 per cent for non-HIV/AIDS HHs; (iii) though remittances form a very small component, they are nevertheless comparatively lower for non-HIV/AIDS HHs at 0.62 per cent, as compared to 2.91 per cent for HIV/AIDS HHs.

The average annual total outflow is a minimum of ₹97,123 per HIV/AIDS HH, with the figure being higher at ₹1,09,514 in case of the control group. Incidentally, the average (wage/non-wage) income per HIV/AIDS HH was only ₹63,126, with the same being higher at ₹1,07,280 for non-HIV/AIDS HHs. This is an indicator that while in case of non-HIV/AIDS HHs average annual HH income is relatively close to the average annual outflow (inclusive of saving/investment), in case of HIV/AIDS HHs the outflow exceeds the total annual HH income substantially; it is just about 0.65 times the size of average annual HH income.[28] It is pertinent to mention that 84.5 per cent of the HIV/AIDS sample HHs had total annual HH income less than the average total annual HH outflow as cited above.

To conclude, HIV infection results in significant additional expenses which poor HHs in particular are least capable of coping with. In urban areas in Côte d'Ivoire, the outlay on school education was halved and expenditure on health more than quadrupled (UNAIDS 2000b, in Adeyi et al. 2001: 10). Even where HIV treatment is free, PLWHA are often subject to bear substantial out-of-pocket expenses to cover transport, tests and medicines not provided for by the public health care providers. In line with the findings of the present study, other studies too recorded the adverse effects that HIV/AIDS has on HHs vis-à-vis expenditures. A study in New Delhi found that due to reasons like doubling of medical expenses, average monthly expenditure of HIV/AIDS HHs exceeded income, with HHs selling assets and spending less on entertainment and education, with 17 per cent of those withdrawing children from school putting them to remunerative activity (ILO 2003, in UNAIDS 2006: 85 and 100). A study in South Africa found that already poor HIV/AIDS HHs were further reducing spending on necessities such as clothing and electricity; with falling incomes forcing about

6 per cent Hhs to reduce expenditure on food, with almost half the Hhs reporting insufficient food (Avert 2008; KFF 2002). In Goa, decreasing incomes and rising expenditures have made HHs to even occasionally disown or abandon expired HIV+ members lying in hospitals and morgues (to be later taken care by state agencies or NGOs) on account of inability to bear expenses on funeral rites.

3.2 How and From Where the Household Rupee Comes

This section is divided into two broad parts: total annual HH income and 'others'; the latter being made up of dissavings, borrowings and UUI.

3.2.1A Household Income

One primary source from where the HH rupee comes from is wage and non-wage income; the latter including among others, pension. With regard to the HIV/AIDS HHs sample, irrespective of their own HIV status, there were 80 widows, 28 (35 per cent) of whom were receiving pension.[29] In continuation to what has already been shown in Chapter 2 (Section 2.1/Table 2.1i) while the average annual total HH income (excluding interest) was ₹63,126 and ₹1,07,280 for HIV/AIDS and non-HIV/AIDS HHs respectively, the annual per capita income was ₹16,750 for HIV/AIDS HHs and ₹23,800 for non-HIV/AIDS HHs members. While wage income per HH was about ₹58,025 and ₹1,04,990 in HIV/AIDS and non-HIV/AIDS HHs respectively, the non-wage component was about ₹5,111 and ₹2,294 respectively.[30]

The distribution of sample HHs based on annual HH income slabs has been shown in Table 3.2.1A. While majority of HIV/AIDS HHs at 64 per cent were clustered in the bottom two slabs of up to ₹50,000, the figure was only 20.5 per cent in case of the control group, with the majority at 71.5 per cent being in the superior

Table 3.2.1A

Comparative distribution of sample HHs based on annual HH income slabs

Income slabs	HIV/AIDS HHs				Non-HIV/AIDS HHs			
	Male-headed	*Female-headed*	*Total HHs*	*% of HHs*	*Male-headed*	*Female-headed*	*Total HHs*	*% of HHs*
Up to ₹25,000	25	32	**57**	**28.5**	1	2	**3**	**1.5**
₹25,001–50,000	35	36	**71**	**35.5**	18	20	**38**	**19**
₹50,001–1,00,000	33	9	**42**	**21**	60	12	**72**	**36**
₹1,00,001–1,50,000	11	3	**14**	**7**	35	8	**43**	**21.5**
₹1,50,001–2,00,000	6	1	**7**	**3.5**	26	2	**28**	**14**
₹2,00,001–2,50,000	1	1	**2**	**1**	5	2	**7**	**3.5**
₹2,50,001–3,00,000	0	0	**0**	**0**	2	0	**2**	**1**
₹3,00,001–5,00,000	5	1	**6**	**3**	5	2	**7**	**3.5**
Above ₹5,00,000	1	0	**1**	**.5**	0	0	**0**	**0**
Total	**117**	**83**	**200**	**100**	**152**	**48**	**200**	**100**

Source: Author's field work.

income slabs ranging from ₹50,001 to 2,00,000. That majority of the PLWHA are from lower economic backgrounds, corresponds to the significant correlation that appears to exist in several parts of the world between HIV prevalence rates and poverty levels/income inequalities (UNESC/ESCAP 2004: 3). Incidentally, not only is the HIV concentrated among the poor, but also the poor having less access to information and health care services, are more likely to be forced by circumstances into making sub-optimal choices (World Bank 1997), with the disease therefore proving harder to tackle among such people (Farmer 1999; both in Bloom et al. 2001a: 8). While poverty contributes to HIV, the latter in turn contributes towards increasing poverty further.

Statistical tests reveal the existence of a *very significant* association as well as differences between gender of the HH head and total annual HH income, wherein it was primarily the female-headed HHs which belonged to HHs with lower incomes. The association/difference was likewise *very significant* for the sample of non-HIV/AIDS HHs as well.

3.2.1B Others

As mentioned earlier, this section covers three broad modes, namely dissavings, borrowings and UUI, which provide resources to HHs over and above the total annual HH income. Although the focus of the present study was on the last one year, nevertheless an overview of resources raised by HIV/AIDS HHs ever since detection of HIV has been outlined herein.

Studies like Bloom et al. (2001b) and Pitayanon et al. (1997) have shown that the socio-economic impact of death due to AIDS is often greater than the costs of diseases or death from other causes, with the cost of treatment/care running for several years and draining HHs savings within a shorter span of time than death on account of other causes (in Nielsen and Melgaard 2004: 43). Pitayanon et al. (1997) highlighted how in Thailand once a member developed AIDS, 60 per cent HHs used savings for medical expenses, 19 per cent sold property and 11 per cent borrowed for treatment and consumption needs (in Narain 2004: 29 and Nielsen and Melgaard 2004: 44). In India as well, studies like those of Pradhan et al. (2006) and Verma et al. (2002) record how HHs resort to borrowings and liquidation of assets due to economic pressures created by HIV/AIDS. As appropriately mentioned by Elizabeth Reid (2000b: 41), poverty caused by HIV-related illness and death deepens existing poverty, creates new poverty and increases indebtedness.

The present study found that the overwhelming majority of 167 (83.5 per cent) HIV/AIDS sample HHs resorted to liquidation/sale of assets and/or borrowings at some point of time or the other ever since HIV detection; that too exclusively because of HIV/AIDS contributed needs. Of the remaining 33 (16.5 per cent) HHs, 10 made use of past savings, with two HHs even resorting to UUI. Considering the above, in all reality therefore, only 21 (10.5 per cent) HIV/AIDS HHs did not resort to sale/liquidation or borrowings in the true sense ever since HIV detection, and managed all HH needs with wage and non-wage income itself. Quite similar to the findings of the present study (see Table 3.2.1B), Pradhan et al. (2006: 94) also found that the borrowings and liquidation of assets was primarily resorted to by those from the lower income brackets,

Table 3.2.1B

Distribution of HHs for total amount raised© since HIV detection and annual HH income

Figures in ₹		Total amount raised since HIV detection excluding UUI and liquidation of bank deposits									
	Nil^	Up to 5,000#	5,001–10,000	10,001–25,000	25,001–50,000	50,001–1 lakh~	1–2 lakhs	2–5 lakhs	5–7.5 lakhs	Above 10 lakhs*	Total
Up to 25,000	0	22	9	11	5	2	6	1	1	0	**57** **28.5%**
25,001–50,000	6	14	8	15	11	11	1	5	0	0	**71** **35.5%**
50,001–1 lakh~	10	7	4	8	4	7	0	1	1	0	**42** **21%**
Annual HH income slabs · **1–1.5 lakhs**	6	1	0	1	0	3	1	1	0	1	**14** **7%**
1.5–2 lakhs	3	0	1	0	1	1	0	0	1	0	**7** **3.5%**
2–2.5 lakhs	1	1	0	0	0	0	0	0	0	0	**2** **1%**
2.5–3 lakhs	0	0	0	0	0	0	0	0	0	0	**0**
3–5 lakhs	4	0	0	0	0	0	1	1	0	0	**6** **3%**

(Table 3.2.1B Continued)

(Table 3.2.1B Continued)

Figures in ₹		Total amount raised since HIV detection excluding UUI and liquidation of bank deposits									
	Nil^	Up to 5,000#	5,001–10,000	10,001–25,000	25,001–50,000	50,001–1 lakh~	1–2 lakhs	2–5 lakhs	5–7.5 lakhs	Above 10 lakhs*	Total
Above 5 lakhs	1	0	0	0	0	0	0	0	0	0	**1** 0.5%
Total	**31** 15.5%	**45** 22.5%	**22** 11%	**35** 17.5%	**21** 10.5%	**24** 12%	**9** 4.5%	**9** 4.5%	**3** 1.5%	**1** 0.5%	**200** 100%

Source: Author's field work.

Notes: ~One lakh is equal to 0.1 million.
@Excluding raising through UUI and liquidation of bank deposits.
*There was no case between ₹7.5 and 10 lakhs and hence the corresponding column has not been kept in the table.
^Includes 10 which actually liquidated bank deposits—the same have not been considered herein.
#Includes 24 HHs whose amounts have been shown herein as ₹1 each…these have resorted to UUI in the last one year itself. These have not been considered for analyses in this sub-section since it deals only with amounts raised through borrowings and sale/liquidation of assets (excluding bank deposits).

with the majority of these incidentally raising funds on the lower side primarily due to poor asset position of the HHs.

Of those HHs which went for sale/liquidation of assets and/ or borrowings since HIV detection, 97.60 per cent resorted to borrowings, 40.72 per cent to sale/liquidation of jewellery,[31] 24.55 per cent to sale/liquidation of bonds/fixed deposit receipts/past savings, 10.18 per cent each to sale/liquidation of HH goods/ vehicles, with 2.99 and 2.40 per cent selling/liquidating house property and agricultural land respectively. Of the 167 HHs which resorted to sale/liquidation of assets and/or borrowings, 81 (48.50 per cent) resorted to two or more of the mentioned modes; while 63 (77.78 per cent) of these resorted to two modes, 15 (18.52 cent) resorted to three, two (2.47 per cent) to four and one (1.23 per cent) to as high as five modes.

The mean amount raised by HHs since HIV was first detected, excluding amounts raised through UUI and liquidation of bank deposits/past savings, was ₹52,354 (SD: 143291) with the maximum amount raised being ₹15,00,000.[32] As Table 3.2.1B shows, 86.98 per cent of the HHs which actually raised resources (89 per cent of the total sample HHs), resorted to sale/liquidation/borrowings (excluding UUI and liquidation of bank deposits) of amounts up to ₹1,00,000 each. It needs to be noted that the amount raised as shown in Table 3.2.1B reflects values on the lower side since a large number of HHs, as shown in a later section, have resorted to UUI in the last one year itself, with a number of HHs also resorting to liquidation of bank deposits (both not considered in Table 3.2.1B); besides 132 HHs which resorted to borrowings and sale/liquidation of assets being unable to recollect accurately the actual amounts raised in earlier years. Seeing the large number of HHs depending on UUI during the last one year itself, one cannot ignore its role in earlier years as well, though with no way of calculating the same on account of its very nature: hidden and unrevealed. Thus, while figures provided in Table 3.2.1B are confirmed ones, the real figures could only be higher than those shown.

Related to amount generated since HIV detection being higher than shown herein is the noting pertaining to the 24 HHs belonging to the raised 'up to ₹5,000' slab (Table 3.2.1B). These are HHs whose details are not available; they have entirely/exclusively depended on UUI. They have been placed in the bottom slab under the assumption that they have raised at least ₹1 each; in reality, they could actually be in higher slabs. Incidentally, if these HHs are dropped (with all other HHs retained even if amount generated were nil), mean amount raised since HIV detection would be higher at ₹59,492 (SD: 151397).[33]

Statistical tests found *no significant* association between gender of the HH head and amount of resources raised since HIV detection (excluding UUI and liquidation of bank deposits); similarly, *no significant* difference was found in amount raised based on gender. The findings are indicators that irrespective of the gender of the HH head, HIV/AIDS HHs had to raise funds since HIV detection for the purpose of coping with HIV/AIDS contributed needs.

3.2.1Ba Dissavings

All the above was with reference to sale/liquidation of assets and borrowings since detection of HIV in the HH. Focusing on only the last one year, since it was the primary objective of the present study, it was found that 72 (36 per cent) HIV/AIDS HHs (47 male-headed and 25 female-headed) had resorted to dissavings involving sale/liquidation of HH assets/property/bank deposits, etc., to generate resources to meet HH expenses and overcome deficits contributed (in)directly by HIV/AIDS (see Table 3.2.1Ba). Incidentally, the corresponding figure was only 25 (12.5 per cent) for non-HIV/AIDS HHs (18 male-headed and seven female-headed) despite these HHs having assets for liquidation/sale, unlike many HIV/AIDS HHs where there were hardly any since the same were already liquidated/sold earlier due to HIV/AIDS related reasons.[34] In terms of mean values, dissavings for all HIV/AIDS sample HHs taken together (₹8,771 per HH) were 1.83 times that for non-HIV/AIDS HHs sample (₹4,790 per HH). Statistical tests found the differences in the amounts dissaved in the two samples to be *very significant* in nature. Incidentally, statistical tests found *absence of significant* association between gender of the HH head and dissavings during the year for HIV/AIDS HHs as well as for non-HIV/AIDS HHs.

Table 3.2.1Ba

Comparative dissavings (including its forms) in the last one year

	HIV/AIDS HHs					Non-HIV/AIDS HHs				
	N	Min (₹)	Max (₹)	Mean (₹)	SD	N	Min (₹)	Max (₹)	Mean (₹)	SD
Amount dissaved in cash	41	2,000	1,24,000	23,537	28,785	22	1,000	2,75,000	40,273	70,163
Sale of jewellery	22	200	60,000	11,614	15,347	4	2,000	50,000	18,000	22,045
Sale of agricultural land	1	36,000	36,000	36,000	–	0	–	–	–	–
Sale of house/flat/plot	2	4,000	3,00,000	1,52,000	209,304	0	–	–	–	–
Sale of other things	18	220	50,000	10,762	15,400	0	–	–	–	–
Total dissavings (concerned HHs only)*	72	200	3,00,000	24,364	41,635	25	1,000	2,75,000	38,320	72,199
Total (all HHs)	200	.00	3,00,000	8,771	27,494	200	.00	2,75,000	4,790	28,108

Source: Author's field work.

Note: *Total number of HHs with dissavings does not correspond with figures given for the various heads of dissavings since some HHs have opted for more than one mode of dissavings.

Similarly, there were *no significant* differences in total dissavings in both samples based on gender. Dissavings were thus gender independent in nature.

An interesting facet related to dissavings brought out by the study was of the 128 (64 per cent) HHs which did not dissave, only 31 (24.22 per cent) had neither borrowings nor UUI during the last one year. Of the rest, 97 (75.78 per cent) had borrowings, UUI or both. This situation arises because in many cases as mentioned, HHs had already exhausted through earlier liquidation/sale most of their savings/assets with hardly any remaining for further dissaving. Of the 97 HHs mentioned, while 22 had only borrowings, 36 had only UUI and 39 had both. The corresponding figure of those who resorted to borrowings, UUI or both, despite there being no dissavings during the year, was only 19 in the case of the non-HIV/AIDS HHs sample, of which three had only UUI, 14 had only borrowings and two had both (for more details see Table 3.2.1Bc[+]ii in Section 3.2.1Bc[+]). Incidentally, relating dissavings to savings for all sample HHs taken together, while in case of the HIV/AIDS HHs sample dissavings were greater than savings by 1.32 times, in case of the non-HIV/AIDS HHs sample, not only were dissavings lower than savings, but also they formed an extremely small portion of the size of savings at 0.19.

3.2.1Bb Borrowings

The adverse financial impact of HIV/AIDS on HHs, particularly on account of high medical expenses, can cause increased indebtedness of HHs (ILO 2003: 32; Pradhan et al. 2006: 59). The present study revealed that 163 (81.5 per cent) HIV/AIDS HHs had resorted to borrowings in some form ever since HIV detection. Of these, while 101 (61.96 per cent) HHs had borrowings during the last one year as well, the remaining 62 (38.04 per cent) did not, though they had done so earlier. Incidentally, 33 (32.67 per cent) HHs which borrowed during the year were alongside making loan repayments. In contrast to the HIV/AIDS HHs, only 28 (14 per cent) non-HIV/AIDS HHs resorted to borrowings during the year of which 22 (78.57 per cent) started loan repayments, with three (13.64 per cent of those making loan repayments) even clearing the loan amount taken. The above shows the relative superior position of non-HIV/AIDS HHs when it comes to numbers of HHs and borrowings.

Almost two-thirds of the HIV/AIDS HHs which borrowed did so from relatives and/or friends, with 3 per cent borrowing from employers and 13.5 per cent borrowing from financial institutions and money-lenders. The vulnerability of HIV/AIDS HHs to fall into the clasp of money-lenders who lend at exorbitant rates of interest arises: (i) since banks are unlikely to lend for meeting HIV/AIDS related expenses; (ii) because of ignorance of many HIV+ members due to the overall background of HHs; and (iii) due to absence of HH assets to provide as security/collateral for availing institutional finance. The present study revealed that borrowing from money-lenders in Goa was usually done at an interest rate of 10 per cent per month.[35]

Of the 101 HIV/AIDS HHs that resorted to borrowings over the course of last one year, while 33 (32.67 per cent) had only borrowings, the remaining 68 (67.33 per cent) had alongside resorted to UUI as well for raising funds. Unlike these high numbers, in case of the control group of the 28 HHs which resorted to borrowings during the year, while there were 23 (82.14 per cent) HHs with borrowings and nil UUI, the number resorting to both was only five (17.86 per cent). Incidentally, while the number of HIV/AIDS HHs from the total sample with nil borrowings and nil UUI during the year were 50 (25 per cent) in case of non-HIV/AIDS HHs the corresponding figure was an overwhelming majority of 166 (83 per cent) HHs.

Table 3.2.1Bb shows that average amount of borrowings, whether for HHs resorting to borrowings or for all sample HHs taken together, is higher in case of the HIV/AIDS HHs sample than the control group. The mean borrowing of all HIV/AIDS HHs taken together was 5.18 times that of non-HIV/AIDS HHs.[36] Statistical tests show the differences in the amount borrowed by the two samples to be *very significant* in nature.

Leaving aside five HHs whose borrowings were largely for reasons such as education and marriage of children, borrowings in the case of majority of the HIV/AIDS HHs were primarily or

Table 3.2.1Bb

Comparative borrowings in the last one year

	HIV/AIDS HHs				Non-HIV/AIDS HHs			
		Min	*Max*	*Mean*			*Min*	*Max*	*Mean*
	N	*(₹)*	*(₹)*	*(₹)*	*SD*	*N*	*(₹)*	*(₹)*	*(₹)*	*SD*
Concerned HHs	101	401	2,70,000	26,647	39,879	28	2,500	1,00,000	18,554	20,505
Total HHs	200	.00	2,70,000	13,457	31,266	200	.00	1,00,000	2,598	9,935

Source: Author's field work.

even exclusively illness driven, directly or indirectly attributable to HIV/AIDS (specifically due to the high medical expenses). In some HHs, while borrowings were used partly for medical expenses and partly for others, a few HHs were borrowing just to alongside pay-off earlier HIV contributed debt; with a number of other HHs borrowing for business or purchase of assets, but diverting the same subsequently towards meeting medical expenses. The diversion of borrowed amount occurs usually in two ways: (i) amount is originally borrowed *ante*-HIV detection for business; post-detection of HIV, the amount is used for taking care of illness related expenses and (ii) since institutional borrowings are not easily available for the needs of PLWHA, including their medical requirements, some HIV+ individuals in desperation occasionally borrow citing business as the reason and later on getting the amount sanctioned divert the same towards meeting illness related expenses. Unlike HIV/AIDS HHs, in case of non-HIV/AIDS HHs, borrowings of the 28 HHs were exclusively or primarily not for medical reasons. Borrowings for medical reasons was resorted only by two (7.1 per cent) HHs; with the remaining seven (25 per cent) borrowing for the purpose of marriage; one each (3.6 per cent each) borrowing for purchase of durable goods, business and education; and the remaining 16 (57.1 per cent) borrowing for 'other' purposes, including combination of reasons.

Statistical tests found *no significant* association between gender of the HIV/AIDS HH head and whether the HH resorted to borrowing during the year. Likewise, there were *no significant* differences in the amount borrowed based on gender in the HIV/AIDS HHs. However, unlike the HIV/AIDS HHs, in case of the non-HIV/AIDS HHs, statistical tests found *very significant* association as well as differences. The results are indicators that while in case of HIV/AIDS HHs, the need for borrowings takes place irrespective of gender of the HH head; in case of non-HIV/AIDS HHs, borrowings are gender dependent, with female-headed HHs being primarily those resorting to borrowings.

3.2.1Bc Unrequited and/or Unrevealed Income (UUI)

One important way, relatively unknown and practically undocumented in literature, how many HHs, especially the lower income bracketed HIV/AIDS HHs, cope with deficits and high expenditures, as revealed by the present study, is through the help of UUI[37]; which among others include unrequited receipts/income and even getting income occasionally through dubious sources such as gambling, prostitution[38] and/or petty offenses/illegalities. Out of the total HIV/AIDS HHs sample, 117 (58.5 per cent) depended on UUI during the last one year, of which details of nine are unknown since all their expenses were fully sponsored by externals such as NGOs and relations. Incidentally, of those who depended on UUI, while 49 (41.88 per cent) HHs had UUI but no borrowings, the remaining 68 (58.12 per cent) had both. In contrast, there were only 11 (5.5 per cent) non-HIV/AIDS HHs depending on UUI during the year; of which while six (54.55 per cent) had only UUI, five (45.45 per cent) had both.

Table 3.2.1Bc shows not only the larger number of HIV/AIDS HHs depending on UUI than the non-HIV/AIDS HHs, but also the high average amount raised via UUI by the concerned HIV/AIDS HHs (that is, those depending on UUI) as well as *all* sample HIV/AIDS HHs taken together. The mean amount raised via UUI by the entire HIV/AIDS sample is 32.49 times the figure of the control group.[39] It needs to be remembered that dependence on UUI is far greater than that shown herein since nine HHs got their needs fully sponsored, besides three others getting additional support besides their own UUI. Statistical

Table 3.2.1Bc

Comparative profile of UUI of the last one year

	HIV/AIDS HHs				Non-HIV/AIDS HHs				
	N	Min (₹)	Max (₹)	Mean (₹)	SD	N	Min (₹)	Max (₹)	Mean (₹)	SD
Concerned HHs	108*	1,000	1,30,000	25,148	22,118	11	3,000	15,500	7,591	4,277
Total sample HHs	200	.00	1,30,000	13,580	20,516	200	.00	15,500	418	1,982

Source: Author's field work.

Note: *Besides the 108 HHs, there were another nine which depended on UUI. They have not been included herein since their details are unknown; all their expenses were fully sponsored by others. Incidentally, among the 108 HHs, there were three which besides having UUI included herein, had additional UUI, details of which are unknown. In reality, therefore, the mean amount generated through UUI would have been higher than shown herein.

tests reveal that the amount raised via UUI by the two samples in the last one year to be *very significantly* different. Incidentally, statistical tests also highlight the existence in both samples of a *very siginificant* association between gender of the HH head and whether resorted to UUI during the year; with figures showing that it is the female-headed HHs which are more dependent on UUI than male-headed ones. Likewise, difference in mean amount of income raised via UUI (on the basis of gender of the HH heads) was found to be also *very significant*.

3.2.1Bc⁺ Borrowings Versus UUI

On account of much dependence of HIV/AIDS HHs on borrowings and UUI, and the important role that the two play, a comparative picture of the two is appropriate (see Table 3.2.1Bc⁺i).

That UUI plays a major role in HIV/AIDS HHs cannot be trivialized in any way. Unlike in case of non-HIV/AIDS HHs, it is UUI that enables numerous HIV/AIDS HHs to literally, survive. It needs to be remembered that HIV/AIDS HHs in general have a low standard of living; lower than their non-HIV/AIDS counterparts on account of various HIV/AIDS contributed compromises. If one

Table 3.2.1Bc'i

Summarized details related to borrowings and UUI

	HIV/AIDS HHs		Non-HIV/AIDS HHs	
	No. of HHs	*Percent of total sample HHs*	*No. of HHs*	*Percent of total sample HHs*
HHs with borrowings last year	101	50.5	28	14
HHs with borrowings as well as UUI last year	68	34	5	2.5
HHs with only borrowings last year and nil UUI	33	16.5	23	11.5
HHs with UUI last year	117	58.5	11	5.5
HHs with only UUI last year and nil borrowings	49	24.5	6	3
HHs exclusively dependent only on UUI last year	9^	4.5	nil	nil
HHs with nil borrowings and nil UUI last year	50	25	166	83
HHs that resorted to borrowings since HIV detection	163	81.5	–	–
HHs which resorted to borrowings earlier but not last year	62	31	–	–
HHs with nil borrowings and nil UUI since HIV detection	30	15	–	–

Source: Author's field work.

Note: ^Their details are unknown since all their needs were fully sponsored; they have not been considered for the purpose of obtaining the mean of the concerned HHs.

excludes the 50 HIV/AIDS HHs having nil borrowings and nil UUI in the last one year; irrespective of whether they had borrowings, UUI or both, the majority of HIV/AIDS HHs at 92 (61.33 per cent) had greater amount generated through UUI than the amount raised through borrowings.[40]

In contrast to the HIV/AIDS HHs sample where there were 150 (75 per cent) HHs having either borrowings, UUI or both during the year, the corresponding figure for non-HIV/AIDS HHs was only 34 (17 per cent). Of these, while seven (20.59 per cent) had UUI greater than borrowings, the remaining 27 (79.41 per cent) had UUI less than borrowings. It is thus obvious that besides the number of HIV/AIDs HHs depending on UUI being higher than non-HIV/AIDS HHs, the percentage of those relying more on UUI as compared to borrowings is also higher in the former. One reason for the extra dependence on UUI in case of HIV/AIDS HHs is that many do not have any collateral or security to offer for the purpose of resorting to borrowing; assets which could have been offered have already been sold or liquidated earlier. Additionally, a comparatively large number of HIV/AIDS HHs are already in debt, with some yet to begin loan repayment. Under these circumstances, generally absent in non-HIV/AIDS HHs, it is UUI that takes primary role (over borrowings) to cover deficits and meet HH expenses. Notwithstanding the fact, as mentioned in the previous section, that there was a significant association between gender of the HH head and dependence on UUI (with the dependence being more on the part of women), there was *no significant* association found between gender and the size of UUI vis-à-vis borrowings[41] for both the study samples.

That borrowings and UUI are important modes of generating resources for HIV/AIDS HHs can be additionally seen from the fact that even those HHs which did not dissave (see Section 3.2.1Ba), actually did opt for borrowings, UUI or both during the year. As the said section revealed, while 97 (75.78 per cent) of the non-dissaving HIV/AIDS HHs resorted to borrowings, UUI or both, the figure for non-HIV/AIDS HHs was only 19—though in percentage terms the figure is 76 per cent considering the small number of HHs involved (details on this class of HHs has been provided in Table 3.2.1Bc[+]ii). Statistical analysis found *no significant* association (in both the samples) between gender of the HH head and whether borrowed during the last one year despite no dissavings; and between gender of the HH head and whether resorted to UUI despite no dissavings. Incidentally, unlike the mentioned absence of significant association, in the case of HIV/AIDS HHs, statistical tests found a *very significant* association between 'whether UUI was

Table 3.2.1Bcⁱii

HHs opting for borrowings, UUI or both during the year despite no dissavings

	HIV/AIDS HHs (N = 90*)				Non-HIV/AIDS HHs (N = 19)			
	Min (₹)	Max (₹)	Mean (₹)	SD	Min (₹)	Max (₹)	Mean (₹)	SD
Borrowings	.00	1,48,000	17,220	27,342	1.00	20,000	8,816	6,834
UUI	.00	90,000	17,584	19,215	.00	15,500	2,158	4,243
Total: Borrowings and UUI	1401	1,48,000	34,804	28,016	2,500	35,500	10,974	7,929

Source: Author's field work.
Note: *Besides these HHs, there are additional seven fully dependent on others. Since their actual UUI are unknown (their borrowings are nil) they are excluded with regard to obtaining the above details.

greater than borrowings' and 'total annual HH income';[42] wherein it was primarily the lower income HHs which had UUI greater than borrowings.[43]

The major role that UUI plays in HIV/AIDS HHs can be seen from another perspective as well. If one compares the various amounts raised by HHs through dissavings[44] and borrowings from the time of detection of HIV (Table 3.2.1B), with and without UUI of the last one year, the difference is as shown in Figure 3.2.1Bc⁺. As can be seen there are relatively a larger percentage of HHs generating a smaller amount, if one excludes amount generated through UUI. However, if one includes UUI, there is a shift in the percentage number of HHs, with there being a greater percentage generating higher amounts. To rephrase the same, before UUI was added, while 49 per cent sample HHs generated resources amounting to 'up to ₹10,000' or none at all; if one adds UUI, the corresponding figure falls to 29 per cent, an indicator of the shift of HHs to higher amount raised. Table 3.2.1Bc⁺iii also shows changes that take place to amount raised since HIV detection when figures of UUI for one year are added. As the table highlights, amount raised by including UUI of one year itself (average ₹65,969 per HH) is 1.26 times the figure as that without UUI (₹52,354 per HH).

Figure 3.2.1Bc⁺

Distribution of HIV/AIDS HHs vis-à-vis revenue raised^ post HIV detection

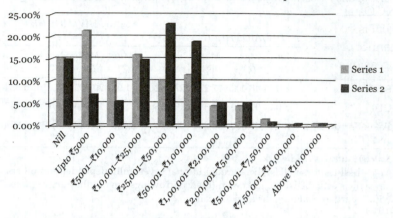

Source: Author's field work.
Notes: Series 1: Percentage of HIV/AIDS HHs before adding UUI of the last one year.
Series 2: Percentage of HIV/AIDS HHs after adding UUI of the last one year.
^Through borrowings and dissavings, but excluding liquidation of bank deposits

Table 3.2.1Bc⁺iii

Amounts raised through dissavings and borrowings^ post HIV detection

	N	Min (₹)	Max (₹)	Mean (₹)	SD
Total amount raised excluding UUI	200	.00	15,00,000	52,354	1,43,291
Total amount raised including UUI of the last one year only	200	.00	15,00,000	65,969	1,46,553

Source: Author's field work.
Note: ^Excluding amount raised through liquidation of bank deposits.

From all of the above it can be safely affirmed that UUI cannot be wished away particularly in the case of HIV/AIDS HHs. Considering their predicaments in not being able to raise funds through gainful employment and/or even borrowings, with HHs becoming impoverished on account of HIV and with HHs having very few assets left for sale/liquidation, it is UUI which plays a major role. And this will continue to be so until alternative arrangements vis-à-vis support are provided by the government, NGOs and/or others. The unfortunate aspect of dependence on UUI is that, while its future availability is very uncertain and hence cannot be depended upon, some modes are unlawful, dubious and occasionally even dangerous, to self and/or others.

3.2.2 Total Inflow

Having seen separately the various ways how and from where the HH rupee comes from, let us now see the sum total of the same; it is this aggregate that helps in understanding how HHs meet their annual requirements.

Table 3.2.2 shows the total amount raised through dissavings, borrowings and UUI during the year. The average amount raised per HIV/AIDS HH is 4.59 times the amount raised by non-HIV/AIDS HHs. Needless to say, statistical results show the difference in amounts raised by the two samples to be *very significant* in nature. As mentioned earlier, amounts raised by HIV/AIDS HHs are primarily or even exclusively on account of reasons contributed by HIV/AIDS (in particular to meet medical needs), unlike the case of non-HIV/AIDS HHs where amounts raised are generally for non-medical purposes.

Figure 3.2.2 highlights how in the case of non-HIV/AIDS HHs much of the HH income (91.22 per cent) comes from wage income itself; unlike HIV/AIDS HHs where the contribution of the same

Table 3.2.2

Comparative total amounts raised through dissavings, borrowings and UUI in the last year

HIV/AIDS HHs (N = 200)				Non-HIV/AIDS HHs (N = 200)			
Min (₹)	Max (₹)	Mean (₹)	SD	Min (₹)	Max (₹)	Mean (₹)	SD
.00	5,00,000	35,803	52,538	.00	3,75,000	7,805	35,006

Source: Author's field work.

Figure 3.2.2

How and from where the HH rupee comes from

HIV/AIDS HHs

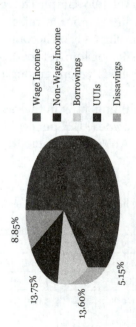

Non-HIV/AIDS HHs

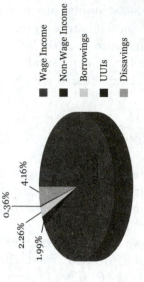

Source: Author's field work.

is comparatively lesser (only 58.68 per cent). This is an indicator that while in the former, the total annual HH income (93.21 per cent) would be more or less close to meeting annual HH needs; in case of the latter it would not, thus making HHs depend much on borrowings and/or UUI. Incidentally, while contribution of borrowings and UUI was as high as 13.60 and 13.75 per cent respectively in HIV/AIDS HHs, the same was only 2.26 and 0.36 per cent respectively in case of the control group.

3.3 Miscellaneous

3.3.1 Modes of Dependence for Assistance

During the course of the study it was found that in the last one year HIV/AIDS HHs met their expenses and plugged existing deficits primarily by depending on modes as shown in Figure 3.3.1. As can be seen majority of the HHs (81 per cent) had to depend on external assistance to cover annual expenses/deficits, with 40 per cent of the total sample depending highly on borrowings/UUI itself. That the role played by borrowings/UUI and even combination

Figure 3.3.1

Modes of dependence of HIV/AIDS HHs for covering expenses/deficits during the year

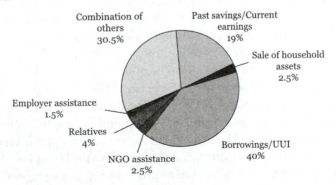

Source: Author's field work.

of mentioned modes (30.5 per cent HHs) was extremely high can be gauged from the fact that while in case of majority of the HHs (80 per cent), NGOs did contribute in providing assistance, the dependence *primarily* on NGOs to cover the annual expenses/ deficits gets reflected as being done by only 2.5 per cent HHs. This is an indication that HHs depended much more on other modes than NGOs. As a consequence of the above, with reference to Figure 3.3.1, finding an HIV/AIDS HH placed in one mode does not mean it does not get assistance from other modes; it only means that the said mode was the *primary* one on which the HH depended upon. Related to the issue of NGOs, it needs to be mentioned that NGOs provide much of the assistance not directly in the form of disbursement of money, but in terms of provisions such as food items/supplements, besides assistance in the form of medical and educational support. If this assistance was absent, expenses/deficits would have been higher than that shown herein as HHs would have had to use own scarce resources, or even stay without enjoying the benefit of some of the basic requirements, thereby worsening living conditions even further.

3.3.2 Provision for Children's Future

The dire straits that HIV/AIDS HHs are in can be additionally seen by the fact that of the HHs with children, over three-fourths (76.5 per cent) made no provision, financial or otherwise, for the future of children. Incidentally, some of these had made some provisions prior to HIV detection, but rising expenses and dwindling income made them use the same subsequently, for example, by liquidating term/recurring deposits and/or selling gold/silver jewellery items. Interestingly, of the remaining 23.5 per cent HIV/AIDS HHs, which claimed to have made provisions for the future of children, while a few made provisions only for one child and not for the other(s), in case of some others, the provisions were more in kind (in case of four HHs, small plots of land which belonged to the HHs even prior to HIV detection, were considered as provisions), with some making provisions which were as paltry as ₹2,000. It needs to be noted that even the so-called provisions are in no way a guarantee that they will ultimately benefit the children, for as seen earlier HHs on account of extreme necessity ultimately make use of the same.

As opposed to the less than quarter of the HIV/AIDS sample HHs, the overwhelming majority of 95.2 per cent non-HIV/AIDS HHs, made provision for their children's future. Statistical tests showed that while there was *no significant* association between gender of the HH head and whether made provisions for the future of children in the case of HIV/AIDS HHs, there was a *very significant* association in case of the control group, the same being to the disadvantage of female-headed HHs. The findings are a reflection that while in case of non-HIV/AIDS HHs, it is the male-headed HHs which usually made provisions for children, with female-headed HHs having a problem on account of financial difficulties experienced post-death of the male-head; in case of HIV/AIDS HHs, difficulties in making provisions are gender independent—they are experienced by male as well as female-headed HHs.

3.3.3 Institutional Assistance

Considering the type and nature of HHs, that the sample HHs in general have practically no scope for availing formal assistance from statutory institutions[45] during the time of need, such as death or medical procedures, can be seen by the fact that only five (2.5 per cent) HIV+ respondents had the benefit of medical insurance, with one discontinuing the same due to financial difficulties. Incidentally, two of those with medical insurance cover had major problems in getting their expenses reimbursed on account of HIV/AIDS. From among the sample respondents, only 28 (14 per cent) had life insurance policy currently in force, with seven others discontinuing their policies on account of poor finances. While none of those who discontinued got back the premium amounts paid (after due deduction of penal charges),[46] of those who currently had a policy in force, some were paying the premium despite immense hardships, through borrowed amounts. Only two respondents from the study sample had the benefit of Employee State Insurance Scheme (ESIS) facility. With majority of HIV/AIDS HHs not covered by the social security or health/life insurance, there is bound to be an adverse long-term effect on savings and asset holdings of HHs (see also Ojha and Pradhan 2006: 3). An observation that came to fore pertaining to life/medical insurance was that, while the same does not contribute much in providing relief to the overwhelming majority of HIV/AIDS HHs, especially since HHs generally do not opt for the same on account of financial difficulties and their overall poor background, there were a few HHs, particularly among the relatively better ones, which though were desirous of making life/medical insurance policies, were denied of the same due to being HIV+.

3.3.4 Disproportionate Burden on Female Members

The present study revealed the presence of relatively more female-headed HIV/AIDS HHs than male-headed HIV/AIDS HHs as compared to the control group where male-headed HHs were more in number (see Appendix I). Incidentally, 20 per cent of the total sample HIV/AIDS HHs comprised of only the mother and children. That female-headed HIV/AIDS HHs, in particular, have greater and disproportionate hardships, at least on certain parameters, has been highlighted in earlier sections herein; with the serious nature of hardships also getting documented by others as well such as Beni (2008); Dixit (2005: 90–91); ILO (2003: 26); Kabir (2008); Pradhan and Sundar (2006); Pradhan et al. (2006); Prasad (2008); Prasad and Somayajulu (2008); UNAIDS (2008: 168); and Xiaoge (2008), who revealed that gender inequalities get further accentuated by AIDS.

In addition to being more susceptible to HIV, women are also relatively more vulnerable to its impact than men (Kadiyala and Barnett 2004: 1891). As the present study and others too have shown, besides most themselves getting infected through their unfaithful husbands, married women are often incorrectly and irresponsibly blamed for the HIV infection of their husbands and/or children (see also Mawar et al. 2005: 475; Singhal and Rogers 2006: 44). The blame game only aggravates the pre-existing depressed socio-economic status of women. Incidentally, on account of the blame game, women often refuse HIV testing because of the difficulties they would encounter (including ostracism and denial of basic economic support) if detected positive; this, in turn, denies them timely and early treatment and presumably a better quality of life[47] (Jain 2008a: 21–22). Though not necessarily arising directly on account of HIV/AIDS but due to the other factors as well, widows (especially younger widows) and their children face greater burden with ownership of lesser assets and distress sales, as well as loss of or threat to tenure status (Aliber et al. 2004: ix–x). Reference to adverse position of women vis-à-vis discrimination and property rights can also be found in Prasad (2008: 48), Reddy (2006: 85) and Roy (2001: 16–17). Reid (2000a: 21) highlights that with growing number of women falling ill and dying, and with those surviving becoming increasingly occupied with caregiving, women have insufficient time for their own children, productive work, self employment or paid work. Incidentally, much of the work performed by women is not quantified monetarily and therefore does not appear in many economic indicators, thus making it difficult to monitor the true macroeconomic impact of the losses despite their serious fallouts (ibid.).

That the generally pre-existing poor economic status of women can only worsen can be fathomed through a quick overview of the situation facing 110 female HIV+ respondents involved in the present study,[48] of which 107 (97.3 per cent) were married. Of these, while the majority (56.9 per cent) were not staying with their husbands or husbands family,[49,50,51] only about 13 per cent got financial support from the husbands (if separated) and/or his family (whether husband was alive or dead), with the majority (72 per cent) being denied right to husband's property by the husbands' family (whether husband was dead or alive).

Notes

1. This helps avoid unnecessarily pointing at UUI and painting a grimmer picture for HIV/AIDS HHs, and at a rosier picture for the control group.
2. It is a different matter that notwithstanding the medical recommendations, the externally appearing high percentage share of HH income spent on food and majority of the HHs getting benefit of partly or fully sponsored food, numerous HHs do make serious compromises vis-à-vis food due to financial difficulties.

3. As income goes up, HHs tend to spend lower percentage of the same on food; and 'substituting' the same with higher spending on non-food items.
4. Minimum amount spent by non-HIV/AIDS HHs on food was ₹1,000.
5. Interestingly, while in the HIV/AIDS HHs sample the minimum amount spent per month on food was nil, the maximum amount was ₹14,000, with the maximum figure being lower at ₹10,500/- in case of non-HIV/AIDS HHs.
6. Some NGOs provide to select HIV+ members a bag of essentials, valued between ₹300 and ₹350 every month, comprising items such as rice, wheat, *dal*, sugar/jaggery, flour, small *Horlicks* bottle, *Dettol* bottle, etc. Some HHs having two or more HIV+ members at times are entitled to more than one bag. In order to alleviate hardships many HIV+ members go to more than one NGO for the free 'bags'.
7. Considering these expenses as those of the HH does not affect the results of the study because the same get reflected under borrowings or UUI.
8. Though there was significant association between gender of the non-HIV/AIDS HH head and 'nature' of food and UUI, the same do not have any substantial bearing overall since very few HHs are involved vis-à-vis the same unlike bigger numbers of HIV/AIDS HHs.
9. Under the broad dual assumptions, confirmed by field observations, that male-heads were generally employed and that usually it is the spouse/woman who heads the HH in the eventuality of death of the male-head/husband.
10. Drop in food consumption due to reasons like lack/fall in appetite due to illness/ongoing medical treatment or bouts of diarrhoea, etc. have not been considered.
11. As a precaution against 'mother to child transmission' (MTCT) of HIV post-delivery, HIV+ mothers are often medically recommended not to breastfeed new born babies.
12. Some NGOs provide nutritional support to only those whose CD-4 count is below a particular minimum.
13. This would result in weakening the immune system further, endangering lives and putting individuals to greater vulnerability to OIs.
14. All hardships cited herein vis-à-vis food is those experienced by the respondents prior to the steep double digit food-inflation which engulfed the nation (Shrinivasan 2010: 13); needless to say, food inflation can only fuel hardships further.
15. In the context of the present study this can happen when women from HIV/AIDS HHs, whether themselves HIV+ or not, may be forced to take up transactional sex to feed their families. If the said women were HIV+, the virus can be transmitted to others; and if the women were HIV negative, they could get the virus from others.
16. Can take place due to the lowering of immunity, compromising of gut and genital mucosal integrity, besides contributing to increasing vertical transmission rates among pregnant and lactating women.
17. Rental amount usually is inclusive of electricity charges.
18. For the purpose of obtaining elementary statistics, while HHs which spent nil amount of their own (even if enjoying the benefit of the concerned item through sponsorship) were excluded, HHs which spent own resources, but later got the same partly/fully reimbursed were included.

19. Some HHs depended exclusively on earnings of the spouse of the male HH head, with the latter, usually HIV+, squandering his entire paltry earnings on alcohol. In some HHs, the sole earning female members had to involuntarily give part of their earnings to the male non-earning HH heads for alcohol.
20. There were more non-HIV/AIDS HHs in self-owned premises than HIV/AIDS HHs.
21. In one HH, with mother and two minor children, the amount spent on toiletries was only ₹20 per month.
22. The same holds good for some other expense heads as well. We need to note that though mean is occasionally higher, the same happens only when we consider the concerned HHs spending money; it generally does not happen if we consider all sample HHs taken together. Thus, on the whole, considering the numbers of HIV/AIDS HHs involved being fewer than non-HIV/AIDS HHs, having higher mean values is not be construed as an indicator of well-being.
23. True even if we trim or ignore a couple of extreme higher-end elements from each sample.
24. The corresponding figure, in terms of per capita per month medical expenses, was nearly four times in the NCAER/NACO/UNDP study (Pradhan et al. 2006: 61).
25. The association/differences were tested at the 0.05 level.
26. Assuming absence of any other claim on the latter from other heads.
27. Pradhan et al. (2006: 60) found medical expenses constituted nearly 11 per cent and 3 per cent of the total consumption expenditure of HIV/AIDS and non-HIV/AIDS HHs respectively.
28. As shown in the next section this gets covered through dissavings, borrowings and/or UUI.
29. Approximately 2/3rd of the widows did not get pension due to reasons such as non-possession of death certificates/ration-cards/other documents, non-cooperation of the late husband's families, lack of awareness, illiteracy, etc.
30. The total annual HH income of HIV/AIDS HHs which is lower than that of the control group is despite the contributions of unmarried joint family members in some HHs. In the highly plausible eventuality that the same may stay separate after their own marriage, the situation for HHs can only worsen.
31. Married women were even compelled to sell their 'precious' *mangalsutras.*
32. If this extreme case is excluded: Mean = ₹45,079; SD = 99994.
33. If the single extreme value mentioned earlier is ignored: Mean = ₹51,261; SD = 105162.
34. Canning et al. (2006a: 14) in another study found 9.9 per cent of the affected HH members selling assets to finance ill health in the preceding year, compared to only 1.5 per cent in the control group.
35. Studies pertaining to sex workers in Sangli (Mahal and Seshu 2000, in Misra et al. 2008: 224) or farmers in Cambodia (Singhal and Rogers 2006: 43) showed that interest charged could even exceed a whopping 100 per cent per month.
36. The figure is 1.44 if one considers only those HHs resorting to borrowings.
37. Resources generated via this source, if at all considered by other studies, possibly get covered in annual HH income or borrowings. UUI, a term coined for the present study, has been excluded from total annual HH income (that

is, wage and non-wage income) and borrowings to get a proper perspective of the role it plays. In the absence of the separation, the *role* would have been lost despite its critical and peculiar nature. Needless to say, while wage/non-wage income is open, certain and 'formal' in nature; UUI is more concealed, uncertain and/or 'informal' in character. Likewise, while borrowings are amounts that have to be repaid with or without interest, UUI is never repaid.

38. The fact, female members (including those who are HIV+) from some HIV/AIDS HHs resort to commercial sex to raise resources to meet fast depleting HH income, was gathered through field interactions (see also Pradhan and Sundar 2006: 106). Incidentally, as available literature unequivocally avers, it is commercial sex workers (CSWs) who are among those most vulnerable to HIV infection in the first place. Though there could be cases to the contrary (to include *ante*-HIV infection non-CSWs resorting to paid sex post-infection due to the need of economic survival), resorting to commercial sex on account of financial necessity by the same women post HIV infection may not be something totally unexpected. In Goa, studies have shown that 0.7 per cent of female urban population was engaged in commercial sex activities (Nair 2009a: 4).

39. If we consider only those HHs which resorted to UUI, the UUI of HIV/AIDS HHs is 3.3 times the size of that of non-HIV/AIDS HHs.

40. Of the rest, while 54 (36 per cent) HHs had UUI less than borrowings, four (2.67 per cent) HHs had both equal.

41. Excluding HHs without UUI and borrowings, and also those where both were equal.

42. Excluding 50 HHs which neither borrowed nor resorted to UUI during the year; and also the four HHs where 'Borrowings = UUI'.

43. Unlike the HIV/AIDS HHs sample, there was *no significant* association in case of the control group.

44. Excluding amounts raised through liquidation of past savings.

45. Like public/private sector insurance companies (where periodic contributions of premium by the insured is mandatory).

46. While three did not do the needful for getting the reimbursement citing 'shame' of showing themselves as the reason, the remaining did not, on account of ignorance.

47. And additionally, not contributing to proper surveillance of the pandemic itself.

48. 64.5 per cent of these belonged to female-headed HHs; majority was HH heads themselves.

49. Majority stopped after the death of the husband, with the remaining stopping ever since husband or self was detected HIV+; with some stopping even before HIV detection for reasons such as harassment, divorce, separation, etc.

50. Break-up of figures of those not staying with husband or his family is as follows: those staying alone or with children, if any: 35.5 per cent; with own parents: 16.8 per cent; with other relatives/friends: 3.7 per cent; at 'Care and Support Homes' arranged places: 0.9 per cent.

51. Of the remaining, while about 31 per cent stayed with husband alone, 12 per cent approximately stayed with husband and/or his family (husband's family in case husband was dead).

4

Health and Medical Expenditure

Health is a priority goal in its own right, as well as a central input to economic development and poverty reduction (Ramani et al. 2008: xiii).

Health and medical expenditures of individuals and HHs on account of HIV/AIDS is an area which has attracted much attention globally on account of its serious nature. While treatment costs of HIV/AIDS are largely unmanageable at the individual level particularly in the developing countries, such countries cannot spare a large amount of resources for prevention/cure; there thus remains a deficit between per capita cost required for prevention/ cure of HIV/AIDS for an economy and per capita expenditure incurred on the same (Sinha 1995: 4). This chapter highlights some newer perspectives vis-à-vis health conditions and medical expenditures of HIV/AIDS HHs. With reference to the comparative analysis involving non-HIV/AIDS HHs, the primary aim was to find if significant differences existed between the two samples despite taking details of *all* members in the age group of 18–60 years from the control group, as opposed to details of *only* the HIV+ respondents in case of the HIV/AIDS HHs sample.

4.1 Introduction

There is a virtuous circle that invariably exists between health and socio-economic development. ADB (2004: 46–47) highlights four key channels through which health affects wealth and economic performance, namely:[1] (i) improved *labour productivity*; according to Weil (2001), health differentials account for 17 per cent of the difference in worker productivity between countries; (ii) positive effect on *education*; an extra year of life expectancy is estimated to increase schooling levels by 0.25 years (Bils and Klenow 2000); (iii) positive effect on *savings/capital accumulation*; and (iv) positive influence on the country's *age structure* through decline in the dependency burden.

HIV/AIDS is a health problem as well as a serious threat to national development. Though not pertaining to HIV/AIDS directly but health in general, India lost $8.7 billion in national income (NI) in 2005 itself due to chronic diseases, with the figure likely to increase to $54 billion in 2015, that is, about 1.27 per cent of India's GDP (Bisserbe 2008: 6). While health problems can condition development, development affects health conditions both positively and negatively. Though development can contribute to the spread of HIV/AIDS through ways such as urbanization and increased mobility of people; economic development generates conditions needed to fight HIV/AIDS, by increasing financial resources, spreading public health systems and/or improving education (UNESC/ESCAP 2004: 4).

HIV/AIDS has been found to make treatment costs disproportionate to the income of affected families. In Sub-Saharan Africa, the direct medical costs of AIDS excluding ART were estimated at about US$ 30 per year per person at a time when public health spending was less than US$ 10 per year for most African countries (UNAIDS 2002, in Avert 2008). In places with high HIV prevalence rates, a large number of hospital beds are found occupied by the infected people. In their study in Nigeria, Canning et al. (2006a) observed that direct health care costs and indirect income loss per HIV+ person were about 32 per cent of the annual income per capita in affected HHs. In Thailand, the cost of treatment of one AIDS person absorbed up to 50 per cent of an average annual HH income (WCC 2002: 98). The findings were similar in India, with figures going as high as 82 per cent in case of low income HHs (Duraisamy 2003, in Nielsen and Melgaard

2004: 44). NCAER/NACO/UNDP in a study involving six Indian states also bring forth the burden that HIV/AIDS bears on HHs, fallouts ranging from medical expenses constituting a high share of total consumption expenditure, to HHs having a relatively lower proportion of expenditure on food; from more dependence of PLWHA on health facilities provided by the government and NGOs for inpatient treatment, to increasing borrowings and liquidation of assets as the stage of infection advances (Pradhan et al. 2006). A study in Delhi estimated ART expenses for a year to be around ₹30,000, with another ₹10,000 for monitoring tests (Over et al. 2004, in Mahal and Rao 2005: 583).

Besides high treatment costs directly related to HIV/AIDS, additional expenses and burdens also cast an intimidating shadow on affected HHs. Out-of-pocket expenses associated with treatment add to the woes. With reference to HIV/AIDS, increased out-of-pocket expenses have been found to arise due to reasons such as absence of insurance benefits, travel fares, food, and non-provision by public health care providers of comprehensive treatment related services including supply of all medicines and poor quality of public services. According to Canning et al. (2006a: 13) out-of-pocket expenses on health care of HIV+ individuals was nearly 32 per cent of the size of per capita income of affected HHs.

Incidentally, the costs of treatment and care fall on those least able to afford these expenses, with the average amount spent by an HIV+ individual in the developing world being between US$5,000 and 12,000 in NPV terms over the course of their life (Drummond and Kelly 2006: 9–10). Kinnon et al. (1994: 12), in their review of a study which presented the principles for calculating the HH demand for health care, indicated that demand is additionally influenced by quality and non-monetary costs. This reflects that accessibility of health care is an important issue. In this context we can state that, while wealthy HHs may or will opt for (expensive) private treatment which could keep infected people asymptomatic for extended periods, the poorest HHs who are forced to rely on public medical provisions will nevertheless have to bear the burden of additional costs, the out-of-pocket costs (Sharma 2006: 122).

Gender disparities vis-à-vis medical treatment has been an area of much concern (see Falleiro and Noronha 2012; Pradhan et al. 2006). Dixit (2005: 134) highlights how in Zambia, though the government was able to reduce the monthly cost of ART from US$64 to US$8 after receiving external/donor support, it was mostly men receiving treatment instead of women, who as per estimates were as high as 70 per cent of the infected population; in one location, of the 40 individuals on treatment, only three were women.

4.2 Total Annual Household Medical Expenditure

Total annual HH medical expenditure represents a sum total of all medical expenditures, inclusive of treatment expenses of all HH members, HIV+ or not; regular monthly medical treatment (RMMT); non-hospitalized illness treatment (NHIT); hospitalized illness treatment (HIT); consultation fees; medical test fees; purchases from pharmacies, etc. Pertaining to the present study, as shown in Table 3.1.1Acii, while mean total annual HH medical expenses for HIV/AIDS HHs were ₹12,991, the same were *very significantly* lower at only ₹2,555 for the control group.

The present study brings out the stranglehold of HIV/AIDS on HHs through its vicious impact on health and medical expenses. For instance, while the total annual HH medical expense as percentage of total 'other annual HH consumption expenditure' (that is, excluding food and regular monthly expenses) was 35.57 per cent for HIV/AIDS HHs, it was only 9.36 per cent for the non-HIV/AIDS HHs (see Table 3.1.1Acii). Also, while total annual HH medical expenditure as proportion of 'total annual HH consumption expenditure' was 13.38 for HIV/AIDS HHs, it was just 2.33 per cent for the control group (see Figure 3.1.2). To highlight the adverse impact of HIV/AIDS on health and medical expenditure from a different perspective, the average 'other annual HH consumption expenditures' *inclusive* of medical expenses which were ₹36,535 per HIV/AIDS HH, become lower at ₹23,544 if medical expenses are *ignored* (see Table 4.2i).[2]

Table 4.2i

Comparative profile of HHs vis-à-vis total 'other annual HH consumption expenditures':^ With and without total annual HH medical expenditures

	With *total annual HH medical expenditures*			Without *total annual HH medical expenditures*		
	Mean (₹)	*Max. (₹)*	*SD*	*Mean (₹)*	*Max. (₹)*	*SD*
HIV/AIDS HHs	36,535	5,47,000	63,491	23,544	4,93,000	47,789
Non-HIV/AIDS HHs	27,311	4,55,000	45,038	23,254	3,34,000	33,729

Source: Author's field work.
Note: ^Excluding food and regular monthly HH consumption expenditures

Table 4.2i shows the adverse position of HIV/AIDS HHs vis-à-vis medical expenses through a comparative analysis involving the control group. The average 'other annual HH consumption expenditure' of non-HIV/AIDS HHs is markedly and significantly lower than that of HIV/AIDS HHs if medical expenses are *included.* Statistical test results show *very significant* difference in total annual HH medical expenditures as well as total 'other annual HH consumption expenditures' for the two samples. Interestingly, the differences with regard to the average values pertaining to the two samples as cited in Table 4.2i, are at best only marginal and insignificant if annual HH medical expenses are ignored. Statistical tests show *no significant* difference in 'other annual HH consumption expenditures' *without* medical expenses pertaining to the two samples. This is indicative of the fact that it is the significant total annual HH medical expense differences that make the two samples to differ from one another. If not for the same, we could confidently say that the two came from the same population.

Table 4.2ii which provides distribution of sample HHs based on 'annual other HH consumption expenditure' slabs, highlights three major aspects with regard to the total annual HH medical expenditure: (i) Medical expenses push-up 'other annual HH consumption expenditures' in both categories of sample HHs—if not for the same there would be more HHs in lower expenditure brackets; (ii) If one *includes* the total annual HH medical expenses, there are relatively more non-HIV/AIDS HHs in lower 'other

Table 4.2ii

Distribution of sample HHs in terms of 'other annual HH consumption expenditure':^ With and without total annual HH medical expenses

Other annual HH consumption expenditure slabs	HIV/AIDS HHs (per cent figures in brackets)		Non-HIV/AIDS HHs (per cent figures in brackets)	
	Inclusive of annual medical expenses	Without annual medical expenses	Inclusive of annual medical expenses	Without annual medical expenses
Up to ₹5,000	14 (7)	38 (19)	19 (9.5)	24 (12)
₹5,001–10,000	28 (14)	44 (22)	46 (23)	55 (27.5)
₹10,001–20,000	53 (26.5)	59 (29.5)	54 (27)	51 (25.5)
₹20,001–30,000	43 (21.5)	28 (14)	40 (20)	32 (16)
₹30,001–50,000	30 (15)	16 (8)	17 (8.5)	18 (9)
₹50,001–75,000	14 (7)	7 (3.5)	13 (6.5)	9 (4.5)
₹75,001–1,00,000	9 (4.5)	1 (.5)	5 (2.5)	5 (2.5)
₹1,00,001–2,00,000	3 (1.5)	3 (1.5)	4 (2)	5 (2.5)
Above ₹2,00,000	6 (3)	4 (2)	2 (1)	1 (.5)
Total	**200 (100)**	**200 (100)**	**200 (100)**	**200 (100)**

Source: Author's field work.
Note: ^Excluding food and regular monthly HH consumption expenditure.

annual HH consumption expenditure' brackets than HIV/AIDS HHs—a reflection of lower medical expenses in general in the former; (iii) Distribution of sample HHs *excluding* the total annual medical HH expenses shows there are generally more non-HIV/AIDS HHs spending higher amount as compared to HIV/AIDS HHs—an indicator of higher spending of the former on non-medical HH consumption items, which usually HIV/AIDS HHs are not capable of due to financial difficulties caused by HIV/AIDS.

Table 4.2iii highlights distribution of sample HHs on the basis of total annual HH medical expenditure slabs. The immense burden that medical expenses bear on HIV/AIDS HHs can be appreciated by seeing that while only a few HHs lie in the lower slabs, with just 4 per cent HHs having nil expenses on account of being illness-free throughout the year (compared to 30.5 per cent in case of non-HIV/AIDS HHs), a relatively large number fall in the higher expense

Table 4.2iii

Distribution of sample HHs on the basis of total annual HH medical expense slabs

	HIV/AIDS HHs				Non-HIV/AIDS HHs			
	Male-headed	*Female-headed*	*Total*	*Per cent of total*	*Male-headed*	*Female-headed*	*Total*	*Per cent of total*
Nil	3	5	8	4	44	17	61	30.5
Up to ₹1,000	19	18	37*	18.5	57	21	78	39
₹1,001–2,500	14	10	24	12	13	3	16	8
₹2,501–5,000	18	12	30	15	10	3	13	6.5
₹5,001–7,500	17	9	26	13	12	3	15	7.5
₹7,501–10,000	8	7	15	7.5	3	0	3	1.5
₹10,001–15,000	10	8	18	9	6	0	6	3
₹15,001–25,000	11	10	21	10.5	5	1	6	3
₹25,001–50,000	9	3	12	6 '	2	0	2	1
₹50,001–1,00,000	6	1	7	3.5	0	0	0	0
Above ₹1,00,000	2	0	2	1	0	0	0	0
Total	**117**	**83**	**200**	**100**	**152**	**48**	**200**	**100**

Source: Author's field work.

Note: *Includes nine HHs whose total annual medical expenses were fully sponsored/reimbursed by others (their expenses are reflected herein as ₹1 since they incurred medical expenses, though not personal; and since they were not free from illnesses during the year).

slabs unlike their counterparts. While 21 per cent HIV/AIDS HHs spent upwards of ₹15,000 on medical expenses, the figure for the control group was only 4 per cent.

Statistical tests reveal *no significant* association between gender of the HIV/AIDS HH head and total annual HH medical expenditure. Likewise, there was *no significant* association between amount of total annual HH medical expenditure and the number of years since HIV was detected. One important implication of the latter is that there are high medical expenses even in HHs where the HIV+ status of respondents was detected 'up to or less than 1 year'. This is primarily on account of two reasons: (i) though the status was detected recently, the infection could have been contracted much earlier and remained unknown (these members may thus not be in the *asymptomatic Stage I* of HIV infection); and (ii) there are other HIV+ members in the HHs whose positive status was detected earlier than that of the respondent.

4.3 Non-hospitalized Illness Episodes/ Treatment (NHIEs/NHIT)

NHIEs for the present study refer to illness episodes of the *last one month* only. NHIEs include those illness episodes which did not necessitate an overnight stay or stay of 24 hours in a hospital/Care and Support Home (C&S Home) but which nevertheless required medical attention, irrespective of whether available, provided, availed of or not.

The study brings to light significant differences in NHIEs with regard to the two study samples; this despite considering illness episodes of *only* the HIV+ respondents (from the HIV/AIDS HHS sample) as compared to *all* HH members from the economically productive age group of 18–60 years from the non-HIV/AIDS HHS sample. While falling immunity levels and being prone to OIs on account of HIV infection itself is the primary cause for being subjected to more illness episodes (both in terms of number of HHs/respondents subjected to illness episodes and number of episodes experienced per respondent) with regard to the HIV/AIDS HHs sample; insufficient access to safe drinking water, sanitation/ toilets, literacy, education, electricity, transport, etc., besides gender inequity have additionally contributed to making sample respondents of HIV/AIDS HHs more vulnerable to infections (see also Panda et al. 2007: 73; Sachs 2008: 3). Much of the NHIEs faced are in HHs belonging to the lower income brackets.

Table 4.3i shows that while 140 (70 per cent) of the non-HIV/ AIDS HHs had no member with NHIEs worth the mention during the course of last one year, the corresponding figure was only 25 (12.5 per cent) with reference to the HIV+ respondents. Similarly, while 58 (29 per cent) HIV+ respondents were either frequently or continuously ill[3] with NHIEs during the last one year, the figure was nil in case of non-HIV/AIDS HHs. During the last one month as well, while 78 (39 per cent) of the total HIV+ respondents were

Table 4.3i

Comparative profile of sample HHs vis-à-vis NHIE/NHIT

	HIV/AIDS HHs		Non-HIV/AIDS HHs	
	Frequency	*Per cent of total sample HHs^*	*Frequency*	*Per cent of total sample HHs^*
Number of times of NHIEs during the last one year				
0	25	12.5	140	70
1	16	8	35	17.5
2	26	13	17	8.5
3	18	9	3	1.5
4	19	9.5	2	1
5 to 10	21	10.5	3	1.5
11 to 20	12	6	0	0
21 and above	5	2.5	0	0
Frequently	37	18.5	0	0
Continuously	21	10.5	0	0
Number of times of NHIEs during the last one month				
0	79	39.5	174	87
1	31	15.5	25	12.5
2	11	5.5	1	.5
3	1	.5	0	0
Frequently	37	18.5	0	0
Continuously	41	20.5	0	0
Number of days ill last month				
2	3	1.5 (2.5)	2	1 (7.7)
3	7	3.5 (5.8)	7	3.5 (26.9)
4	6	3 (5)	4	2 (15.4)
5	6	3 (5)	5	2.5 (19.2)
6–7	4	2 (3.3)	2	1 (7.7)
8–10	11	5.5 (9.1)	4	2 (15.4)
Above 11	6	3 (5)	2	1 (7.7)
Frequently	37	18.5 (30.6)	0	0
Continuously	41	20.5 (33.9)	0	0
Sub-total	*121*	*60.5 (100)*	*26*	*13 (100)*
Those not sick	79	39.5	174	87
Total	**200**	**100**	**200**	**100**

Source: Author's field work.

Note: ^Figures in brackets are approximate percentage figures in terms of said categories only.

frequently or continuously ill, the figure was nil in case of non-HIV/AIDS HHs. Though 175 (87.5 per cent) HIV+ respondents were ill with NHIEs during the last one year, only 121 (60.5 per cent of the total sample or 69.14 per cent of those sick during the year) were ill during the last one month. In contrast, in case of the control group, while 60 (30 per cent) HHs had members who were sick during the year, only 26 HHs (13 per cent of the total sample) had members who were sick during the last one month. Leaving aside those who were ill frequently or continuously during the last month, the average number of days of illness was 6.58 for HIV+ respondents and a lower figure of 5.54 days for members of non-HIV/AIDS HHs (see Table 4.3ii).

Of those subject to NHIEs during the course of the last one month, while almost a quarter of the HIV+ respondents did not seek treatment;[4] the corresponding figure for non-HIV/AIDS HHs was around 19 per cent (Table 4.3iii). Though the latter may still appear as a substantial figure, it is not, considering that it refers only to five HHs, that too by taking details of *all* HH members (18–60 years) and by noting that these did not take treatment not because of the financial difficulties, but because the illness was not considered as serious. In case of the HIV/AIDS HHs though, not seeking treatment was primarily on account of financial inadequacies; and this despite treatment (consultation, medicines and often clinical tests as well) being provided free by the government; with those ill primarily having to incur treatment associated out-of-pocket expenses only, including those related to transport and clinical tests/medicines not provided by the government.

Table 4.3ii

Comparative number of days sick last month excluding those frequently/continuously sick

HIV/AIDS HHs (N = 43)				Non-HIV/AIDS HHs (N = 26)			
Min	*Max*	*Mean*	*SD*	*Minimum*	*Maximum*	*Mean*	*SD*
2	15	6.58	3.95	2	15	5.54	3.48

Source: Author's field work.

Table 4.3iii

Comparative profile of sample HHs vis-à-vis treatment to those sick in the last month

	HIV/AIDS HHs		Non-HIV/AIDS HHs	
	Frequency	*Percentage (concerned HHs only)*	*Frequency*	*Percentage (concerned HHs only)*
Did you seek treatment last month				
Yes	91	75.2	21	80.8
No	30	24.8	5	19.2
Total	121^	100	26	100
If no treatment, reason why				
Illness not considered serious	0	0	5	100
No doctor willing to treat	1	3.3	0	0
Financial constraints	8	26.7	0	0
Lack of time/long waiting	2	6.7	0	0
Ignorance	1	3.3	0	0
Doctor not prescribing any treatment	1	3.3	0	0
Others*	17	56.7	0	0
Total	30	100	5	100
Those who took treatment last month, source of treatment				
PHC/CHC	4	4.4	1	4.8
Government hospital	55	60.4	5	23.8
Private doctor/clinic	21	23.1	15	71.4
NGO	7	7.7	0	0
Others	4	4.4	0	0
Total	91	100	21	100

Source: Author's field work.

Notes: ^While 26 (21.5 per cent) were salary earners, 23 (19 per cent) wage earners and 12 (9.9 per cent) self employed; the remaining 60 (49.6 per cent) were currently not employed. If we consider only the 78 respondents who were continuously/frequently ill, while 11, 14 and four were salary earners, wage earners and self-employed respectively; the majority of 49 were currently not employed.

* Includes combination of cited reasons besides being 'fed-up' of the situation; these at best take only home remedy.

Of those seeking treatment, majority of over 60 per cent HIV+ respondents went to government hospitals (see Table 4.3iii). The figure becomes 72.5 per cent if we add alongside those going to NGOs and Primary/Community Health Centres (PHC/CHC); with the figure becoming almost 77 per cent if all non-private treatment seekers are clubbed together. Unlike HIV/AIDS HHs, in case of non-HIV/AIDS HHs, the majority at over 71 per cent opted for private treatment. Pertaining to HIV/AIDS HHs, while 12 male and nine female HIV+ respondents opted for private treatment, 24 male and 46 female respondents went for non-private treatment primarily provided by the government and NGOs. Statistical tests show *quite significant* association between source of treatment and gender of the HIV+ respondent, with female HIV+ respondents primarily availing government/NGO provided *free* treatment and male respondents opting relatively more for *paid* private treatment.

Pertaining to those ill with NHIEs during the period of last one month, statistical tests found *no significant* association between whether took treatment and gender of the HH head in both the samples. Likewise, there was *no significant* association vis-à-vis gender of the HIV+ respondents and whether those ill went for treatment. Unlike the above, pertaining to the number of years since HIV was detected and whether the HIV+ respondents opted for treatment for NHIEs during the last month, there was *quite significant* association. As can be seen from Table 4.3iv, the ratio of those seeking treatment is higher as the number of years since HIV detection goes on increasing. While 66.66 per cent of those whose HIV+ status was detected '1 year or less' opted for treatment, the

Table 4.3iv

NHIT and number of years since detection of HIV

	Number of years back since HIV was first detected			
	1 year or less	*1 year to 5 years*	*Over 5 years*	*Total*
Yes, took treatment	20	52	19	91
No, did not seek treatment	10	19	1	30
Total	**30**	**71**	**20**	**121**

Source: Author's field work.

figures were higher at 73.24 per cent and 95 per cent for those whose status was found in the range of '1–5 years', and 'over 5 years' (earlier) respectively. Field interactions revealed that the primary reason why there were relatively more HIV+ respondents without treatment whose HIV status was detected ' ≤ 1 year' was that[5] these wanted to keep their HIV+ status under total wraps due to stigma and discrimination. Additionally, many of these were in the state of *denial*. As the number of years since HIV detection goes increasing, relatively more opt for treatment, the primary reasons for the same being: (i) respondents crossing the state of denial and moving into the state of *acceptance* and *hope*; (ii) need for proper and timely treatment being rightly appreciated and understood; and (iii) to ease the relatively more frequent and serious fallouts caused by illnesses/OIs, which in general happen on account of gradual progression in the four stages of HIV leading to AIDS.[6] Leaving aside the issue whether treatment was opted or not, pertaining to the issue of OIs[7] and illness episodes which keep on increasing as the stage of infection increases (and which generally happens as years since HIV detection keeps increasing), it needs to be noted that even with regard to those detected positive '≤1 year', there are still a large number of cases of illness episodes experienced. This is because though the HIV+ status was detected only recently, they could nevertheless have been infected much earlier and hence presently not be in the *asymptomatic Stage I* of infection (see also Pradhan et al. 2006: 118).

If instead of considering all those ill with NHIEs during the last month, we take only the 78 HIV+ respondents who were frequently or continuously ill (see Table 4.3i), about 28 per cent did not go for any treatment (Table 4.3v). The mean age of those continuously/ frequently sick was 36.09 years (SD: 9.31) with the youngest being only 20 years and the oldest 60 years.[8]

Statistical tests showed *no significant* association between gender of the continuously/frequently ill HIV+ respondents and whether took treatment for NHIEs last month. However, unlike the same, there was *quite significant* association between whether those continuously/frequently sick last month took treatment and gender of the respondents' HH head; as well as with the number

Table 4.3v

NHIT of those frequently or continuously sick in the last month

	Male- headed HHs	Female- headed HHs	Total no. of HHs	Per cent of concerned HHs
Went for treatment	26	30	56	71.8
Did not seek treatment	15	7	22	28.2
Total	41	37	78	100

Source: Author's field work.

of years since HIV was detected. Interestingly, unlike most cases where there was either absence of gender of the HH head related association, or if present it was to the disadvantage of female-headed HHs, the present findings show that it is the female-headed HHs which opted more for treatment for continuously/frequently experienced NHIEs (see Table 4.3v). Notwithstanding that further in-depth analysis will have to be done to confirm the said association, especially since the significance was not very strong, field observations nevertheless revealed that female-headed HHs more often than not seek treatment since it is the female-heads in such HHs who are usually HIV+ and it is these who have to take care of the entire HH inclusive of minor/dependent children. With regard to the significant association found vis-à-vis treatment of those continuously/frequently sick and number of years since HIV was detected, the association takes place for reasons similar to those mentioned earlier with regard to those who were ill with NHIEs during the last one month. As was the case earlier, as number of years since detection increase, the numbers of those seeking treatment keep increasing (Table 4.3vi).

Notwithstanding the earlier examples highlighting the adverse position of HIV/AIDS HHs vis-à-vis NHIE/NHIT, Tables 4.3vii and 4.3viii provide additional insight into hardships faced. As can be seen HIV/AIDS HHs face a substantial disadvantage as compared to non-HIV/AIDS HHs, both in terms of numbers of HHs involved and with regard to mean values; and this despite: (i) details of *only one* respondent being considered in the former as opposed to *all* in the 18–60 years age group in the latter; and

Table 4.3vi

Treatment of those frequently/continuously ill with NHIE and years since HIV detection

	Number of years since HIV was first detected			
	1 year or less	*1 year to 5 years*	*Over 5 years*	*Total*
Took treatment	13	32	11	**56**
Did not seek treatment	8	14	0	**22**
Total	**21**	**46**	**11**	**78**

Source: Author's field work.

Table 4.3vii

Comparative figures on duration of NHIT and days bedridden and not gone for work

	HIV/AIDS HHs					Non-HIV/AIDS HHs				
	N	*Min*	*Max*	*Mean*	*SD*	*N*	*Min*	*Max*	*Mean*	*SD*
Duration of treatment (days)*	91	2	30	18.31	10.87	21	3	30	8.29	6.51
No. of days bedridden	28	2	30	13	9.82	2	4	7	5.5	2.12
No. of days not gone for work	28	1	30	17.21	11.86	14	1	30	8.5	7.65

Source: Author's field work.
Note: *Excluding those who took only home remedy and including those whose expenses were fully reimbursed by others.

(ii) majority from the former opting for *free* treatment provided by government/NGOs, with the latter opting more for *paid* private treatment.

In terms of the duration of treatment, number of days bedridden and number of days not gone for work, the figures for HIV/AIDS HHs are more than twice the size of that of non-HIV/AIDS HHs (Table 4.3vii). With regard to expenses, leaving aside transport costs where figures for both the samples are close to each another, while in case of (consultation) fees/medicines the amounts spent by HIV/AIDS HHs were about 3.23 times the size of expenses of non-HIV/AIDS HHs, total average expenses on NHIT of only the concerned HIV/AIDS HHs (that is, those which experienced

NHIEs during the last month, opted for treatment, and incurred some personal/HH expenses on the same) was 2.6 times the size of that of the control group, with the mean total expenditures on NHIT for the entire sample being a whopping 9.8 times higher in the former. Things could only get worse if those who presently got their expenses fully reimbursed by others (not part of Table 4.3viii) did not get the benefit and instead had to incur personal expenses.

Distribution of the total sample HHs based on total expenses incurred on the NHIT during the last one month has been shown in Table 4.3ix. There was *no significant* association/difference found between the same and gender of the HIV/AIDS HHs' heads (similar was the case with the control group). Likewise, there was *no significant* association/difference between the total NHIT expense slabs of the last month and gender of the HIV+ respondents.

Table 4.3viii

Comparative figures of NHIT expenses of sample HHs of the last one month

	HIV/AIDS HHs					Non-HIV/AIDS HHs				
	N	Min	Max	Mean	SD	N	Min	Max	Mean	SD
Amount spent on fees/medicines (₹)*	75	30	1,00,000	2,682	11,589	23	10	5,000	830	1,037
Amount spent on clinical tests (₹)	13	50	10,000	1,064	2,696	5	100	2,000	650	773
Transport costs (₹)	75^	30	2,000	264	331	8	25	1,000	216	328
Total expenditure for concerned HHs (₹)	87^^	30	1,12,000	2,699	12,059	23**	10	8,000	1,046	1,627
Total expenditure of all HHs (₹)	200	.00	1,12,000	1,174	8,040	200	.00	8,000	120	636

Source: Author's field work.
Notes: *Includes those not seeking treatment but who nevertheless made use of home remedy/self-prescribed treatment and who therefore had to spend some nominal amount to get the medicines. The figures do not include those whose expenses were fully reimbursed by others.
**Includes two on home remedy/self-prescribed treatment who had to spend some amount on the same.
^Excluding five HHs whose travel expenses were fully reimbursed by others.
^^Excluding four HHs whose expenses were fully reimbursed by others.

Table 4.3ix

Distribution of sample HHs in terms of total expenses on NHIT in the last one month

	HIV/AIDS HHs				Non-HIV/AIDS HHs			
Expense slabs	Male-headed	Female-headed	Total HHs	Per cent of total HHs	Male-headed	Female-headed	Total HHs	Per cent of total HHs
Nil	68	41	109	54.5	134	43	177	88.5
Up to ₹100	4	4	8	4	3	1	4	2
₹101–250	5	8	13	6.5	3	1	4	2
₹251–500	11	7	18	9	2	0	2	1
₹501–750	7	8	15	7.5	1	2	3	1.5
₹751–1,000	4	2	6	3	3	1	4	2
₹1,001–1,500	8	2	10	5	2	0	2	1
₹1,501–2,500	5	6	11	5.5	3	0	3	1.5
Above ₹2,500	5	5	10	5	1	0	1	.5
Total	**117**	**83**	**200**	**100**	**152**	**48**	**200**	**100**

Source: Author's field work.

A common implication of the above is that HIV/AIDS has adverse bearing on HHs vis-à-vis medical expenditure, irrespective of the gender of the HH head and gender of the HIV+ respondent.

As with total annual HH medical expenditure, HIV/AIDS has a significant adverse bearing with regard to NHIT itself, with statistical analysis showing *highly significant* difference in total NHIT expenses of the last month in the two categories of sample; and this as mentioned earlier despite: (i) NHIT details of *only* the HIV+ respondents being considered, as opposed to details of *all* HH members (18–60 years age group) in case of the control group and (ii) over two-thirds of the treatment availing sample HHs (see Table 4.3iii) opting for the relatively cheaper government/PHC/NGO treatment (occasionally availed free or even fully sponsored), unlike non-HIV/AIDS HHs majority of which at over 71 per cent on experiencing illness episodes opted for the relatively expensive private treatment. That NHIT expenses have a far greater economic impact on HIV/AIDS HHs can be additionally gauged in the proper perspective by realizing that even if expenses of those below 18 and above 60 years are alongside also considered for the control group, the same are still *very significantly* higher in case of the HIV/AIDS Hhs.

Considering the composition of sample HIV/AIDS Hhs, most of those subject to NHIT during the last month came from Hhs belonging to lower total annual income slabs (see Table 4.3x). About 51.6 per cent of the Hhs from the bottom two slabs (that is, up to ₹50,000) bore NHIT expenses, with the figures going up if those not seeking treatment are included. Incidentally, of those who spent nil amounts and who happened to be from the lower annual HH income slabs, a total of 30 HIV+ respondents were actually subject to NHIEs but did not seek treatment primarily due to financial problems; with majority of these at 22 (73.33 per cent) being sick even frequently or continuously.[9]

Situation of HIV/AIDS Hhs vis-à-vis total NHIT expenses can get worse than that portrayed if those sick that have not availed of treatment take recourse to the same and if expense details of other HH members, including the HIV+, are alongside also considered. Additionally, economic impact vis-à-vis NHIEs can worsen further, if besides the direct adverse impact on medical expenses, a thought is also given to the indirect impact, an example in point being the loss of income due to wage-cuts or loss of employment due to illness and/or caregiving.

4.4 Hospitalized Illness Episodes/ Treatment (HIEs/HIT)

Unlike NHIEs which pertained to the *last one month* only, HIEs pertain to illness episodes during the *last one year*. As with NHIEs in the case of HIEs as well, while the sum total episodes of *only* the HIV+ respondents have been considered in case of HIV/AIDS Hhs, it was details of *all* members in the age group of 18–60 years in case of the control group. For the purpose of the present study, HIE/ HIT means illness episodes/treatment that required an overnight or 24- hour stay in a public/private hospital or C&S Home.

Table 4-3x

Distribution of sample HIV/AIDS HHs based on total NHIT expense and annual HH income

All figures in ₹	Total NHIT expenditure slabs								Total
	Nil	Up to 100	101–250	251–500	501–1,000	1001–1500	1,501–2,500	Above 2,500	
Total annual HH income slabs									
Up to 25,000	24*	4	6	5	9	2	4	3	57 (28.5%)
25,001–50,000	38**	2	6	7	7	5	3	3	71 (35.5%)
50,001–1 lakh^	26***	1	0	5	4	3	2	1	42 (21%)
1–1.5 lakhs	10****	0	1	1	1	0	1	0	14 (7%)
1.5–2 lakhs	6	0	0	0	0	0	0	1	7 (3.5%)
2–2.5 lakhs	1	0	0	0	0	0	0	1	2 (1%)
2.5–3 lakhs	0	0	0	0	0	0	0	0	0
3–5 lakhs	4	0	0	0	0	0	1	1	6 (3%)
Above 5 lakhs	0	1	0	0	0	0	0	0	1 (0.5%)
Total	109 (54.5%)	8 (4%)	13 (6.5%)	18 (9%)	21 (10.5%)	10 (5%)	11 (5.5%)	10 (5%)	200 (100%)

Source: Author's field work.

Notes: ^One lakh is equal to 0.1 million.

*Includes 10 who did not opt for treatment despite presence of NHIEs last month.

** Includes 13 who did not opt for treatment despite presence of NHIEs last month.

*** Includes six who did not opt for treatment despite presence of NHIEs last month.

**** Includes one who did not opt for treatment despite presence of NHIEs last month.

A World Bank study had shown earlier that a typical adult
AIDS patient has 17 illness episodes requiring 280 days of care;
20 per cent in hospital (Rao 2000b: 494). The present study
highlights that majority of the HIV+ respondents at 78 per cent
were hospitalized some time or the other since HIV detection (see
Table 4.4i), this despite numerous instances where urgent medical
procedures were indefinitely kept on hold for even up to three years
due to lack of finances. While about 39 per cent of these were
hospitalized only once since HIV detection, an exceptional case
was hospitalized as high as 30 times. Statistical testing has shown
no significant association between whether ever hospitalized after
HIV detection and: (i) gender of the HH heads; (ii) gender of the
HIV+ respondents; and (iii) number of years since HIV detection.

Table 4.4i

Hospitalization details of HIV+ respondents including number of times hospitalized

	No. of HIV+ respondents	Percentage figures
Whether hospitalized ever since detection of HIV		
Yes	156	78
No	44	22
Total	200	100
Number of times hospitalized since detection of HIV		
1	61	39.1
2	34	21.8
3	19	12.2
4	15	9.6
5	7	4.5
6–7	7	4.5
8–10	5	3.2
11–15	4	2.6
16–20	3	1.9
Above 20	1	.6
Total	156	100

Source: Author's field work.

The average number of times being hospitalized for the concerned respondents was 3.29 (SD: 4.10).

Of the 156 HIV+ sample respondents hospitalized since HIV detection, 125 (80.1 per cent) were hospitalized during the course of the last one year. From the point of view of the total HIV/AIDS sample, the said figures represent 62.5 per cent of the respondents. In case of the total non-HIV/AIDS HHs' sample, the corresponding figure was as low as 18 (9 per cent). While 63 (50.4 per cent) HIV+ respondents who were hospitalized, were admitted two or more times during the course of the last one year, the corresponding figure was only two (11.1 per cent) in case of non-HIV/AIDS HHs (see Table 4.4ii). As in case of NHIT where majority of the HIV+ respondents opted for non-private treatment, with regard to HIT

Table 4.4ii

Comparative profile of sample HHs vis-à-vis HIE/HIT

	HIV/AIDS HHs		Non-HIV/AIDS HHs	
	Frequency	*Percentage of total sample HHs^*	*Frequency*	*Percentage of total sample HHs^*
Number of times of hospitalized during the last one year				
1	62	31 (49.6)	16	8 (88.9)
2	31	15.5 (24.8)	2	1 (11.1)
3	14	7 (11.2)	–	–
4	8	4 (6.4)	–	–
5	4	2 (3.2)	–	–
6–7	3	1.5 (2.4)	–	–
8–10	3	1.5 (2.4)	–	–
Sub-total	*125*	*62.5 (100)*	*18*	*9 (100)*
Those not hospitalized last year	75	37.5	182	91
Source of hospitalized treatment last year				
Government hospital	37	18.5 (29.6)	11	5.5 (61.1)
Private	9	4.5 (7.2)	7	3.5 (38.9)
NGO/C&S Home	51	25.5 (40.8)	–	–

(Table 4.4ii Continued)

(Table 4.4ii Continued)

	HIV/AIDS HHs		Non-HIV/AIDS HHs	
	Frequency	Percentage of total sample HHs^	Frequency	Percentage of total sample HHs^
Combination of C&S Home and government hospitals	28	14 (22.4)	–	–
Sub-total	*125*	*62.5 (100)*	*18*	*9 (100)*
Those not hospitalized last year	75	37.5	182	91
Primary source of financing hospitalization expenses last year				
Past savings/present money	46	23 (36.8)	12	6 (66.7)
Employer reimburses	5	2.5 (4)	–	–
Liquidation of assets	3	1.5 (2.4)	1	.5 (5.6)
Borrow from friends/relatives	47	23.5 (37.6)	4	2 (22.2)
Borrow from money lenders/financial institutions	7	3.5 (5.6)	–	–
NGO support	2	1 (1.6)	–	–
Others#	15	7.5 (12)	1	.5 (5.6)
Sub-total	*125*	*62.5 (100)*	*18*	*9 (100)*
Those not hospitalized last year	75	37.5	182	91
Total	**200**	**100**	**200**	**100**

Source: Author's field work.
Notes: ^Figures in brackets are percentage figures of concerned respondents/HHs subject to HIEs only.
#Including combination of earlier cited ways.

as well the overwhelming majority at 92.8 per cent opted for non-private treatment, which among others included treatment in government hospitals, C&S Homes or both. It needs to be noted that, while relatively more opted for private treatment vis-à-vis NHIEs, the number goes down in case of HIEs on account of the prohibitive expenses in private hospitals and lack of access to health insurance (see also Pradhan et al. 2006: 125–126). Unlike the small figure of 7.2 per cent HIV+ respondents who took private HIT, the corresponding figure was much higher at 38.9 per cent in case of the control group. While majority of the non-HIV/AIDS HHs subject to HIEs last year at 66.7 per cent bore the HIT expenses with their own resources (that is, present income and/or past savings), the corresponding figure for HIV/AIDS HHs was only 36.8 per cent.[10] Leaving aside the small number resorting to liquidation of assets, that is, dissavings, there were substantially a large number of HIV/AIDS HHs depending on other 'external' sources for meeting HIT expenses, with a big number of 43.2 per cent depending on borrowings, from relatives and friends, as well as financial institutions and money-lenders (see Table 4.4ii).[11]

Tables 4.4iii and 4.4iv provide a comparative description pertaining to those hospitalized during the course of the last one year; unsurprisingly, HIV+ respondents are at a disadvantage in all respects. For instance, with regard to the total number of days hospitalized during the last one year, while the average was close to a month at 27.08 days in case of the HIV+ respondents, it was only 6.72 days in case of the control group; the former thus had hospitalization days over four times that of the latter, with presently working members thus tending to lose much more in terms of earnings lost in HIV/AIDS HHs.[12] In case of number of times hospitalized in the last one year, while the mean was 2.11 times in case of the HIV+ respondents, it was almost half at 1.11 for the control group. Even here, that the adversity faced

Table 4.4iii

Comparative figures of number of times and days hospitalized in the last one year

	HIV/AIDS HHs (N = 125)				Non-HIV/AIDS HHs (N = 18)			
	Min	*Max*	*Mean*	*SD*	*Min*	*Max*	*Mean*	*SD*
Total no. of times hospitalized last year	1	10	2.11	1.69	1	2	1.11	0.32
Total no. of days hospitalized last year	1	180	27.08	29.91	2	16	6.72	3.91

Source: Author's field work.

Table 4.4iv

*Comparative figures of hospitalization expenses of sample HHs of the last one year^*

	HIV/AIDS HHs				Non-HIV/AIDS HHs				
	N	Min	Max	Mean	SD	N	Min	Max	Mean	SD
Room-rent/ tests/surgery (₹)	69*	200	1,43,000	10,069	22,640	18	200	15,000	5,339	4,863
Transport costs (₹)	117**	50	10,000	562	1,000	14	50	1,000	382	276
Diet/lodging of caregivers (₹)	46	100	9,000	1,564	1,558	7	200	400	264	75
Total hospitalization expenses (₹)	117**	50	1,62,000	7,115	19,494	18	350	15,500	5,739	4,813
Total expenses of all sample HHs (₹)	200	.00	1,62,000	4,162	15,293	200	.00	15,500	517	2,166

Source: Author's field work.
Notes: ^First four rows provide figures of only the concerned respondents/HHs incurring hospitalization related expenses.
*Excluding one respondent whose expenses were totally sponsored by others.
**Excluding eight respondents' expense details since the same were fully sponsored by others.

by HIV+ respondents is greater than what the figures appear to show, can be judged in a more appropriate manner by realizing that there were more hospitalized HIV+ respondents at 125, as opposed to only 18 in case of the non-HIV/AIDS HHs.

Pertaining to HIT expenses (Table 4.4iv), whether with reference to numbers of respondents/HHs involved or actual expenses, the figures pertaining to HIV+ respondents are substantially higher. For example, if we consider the entire sample, the mean total HIT expenses per HIV/AIDS HH standing at ₹4,162 per annum, is over eight times larger than that of the control group where the corresponding figure was only ₹517; and this difference is despite a relatively larger number of the former opting for non-private treatment and considering HIT details of only the HIV+ respondents (unlike details of *all* within 18–60 years in case of the control group). On the expense front, things could have got worse for HIV/AIDS HHs had some respondents not availed the benefit of full/part reimbursement of HIT expenses.[13]

The comparative distribution of sample HHs based on the total HIT expense slabs for the last one year has been provided in Table 4.4v. Statistical tests show *no significant* association/difference existing between the total HIT expenses of sample HIV/AIDS HHs and: (i) gender of the HH head; and (ii) gender of the HIV+ respondent.

Tables 4.4v and 4.4vi reveal that the biggest chunk of 24.5 per cent of the total sample HHs had to bear 'up to ₹500' as total HIT expenses during the course of last one year (the figure gets higher at 39.2 per cent if we ignore those not subjected to HIEs). Close to 74 per cent of the HIV+ respondents belonging to the 'up to ₹25,000' per annum total HH income bracket were subject to HIT last year, with the figure becoming about 69.5 per cent if we include

Table 4.4v

Comparative total HIT expense slabs of sample HHs in the last one year

	HIV/AIDS HHs				Non-HIV/AIDS HHs			
Expense slabs	Male-headed HHs	Female-headed HHs	Total HHs	Percent of total HHs	Male-headed HHs	Female-headed HHs	Total HHs	Percent of total HHs
Nil	43	32	75	37.5	135	47	182	91
Up to ₹500	28	21	49	24.5	1	0	1	.5
₹501–2,500	14	13	27	13.5	4	1	5	2.5
₹2,501–5,000	10	5	15	7.5	4	0	4	2
₹5,001–7,500	5	4	9	4.5	2	0	2	1
₹7,501–10,000	4	0	4	2	2	0	2	1
₹10,001–15,000	3	6	9	4.5	3	0	3	1.5
₹15,001–25,000	4	2	6	3	1	0	1	.5
₹25,001–50,000	4	0	4	2	0	0	0	0
₹50,001–1,00,000	0	0	0	0	0	0	0	0
Above ₹1,00,000	2	0	2	1	0	0	0	0
Total	**117**	**83**	**200**	**100**	**152**	**48**	**200**	**100**

Source: Author's field work.

Table 4.4vi

Distribution of HIV/AIDS HHs sample based on total annual HIT expenses and HH income

			Total HIT expenditure slabs					
	Figures in ₹	*Nil*	*Up to 500*	*501– 2,500*	*2,501– 5,000*	*5,001– 10,000*	*10,001– 50,000*	*Above 50,000*	*Total*
	Up to 25,000	15	16	10	4	4	7	1	**57** **(28.5%)**
	25,001– 50,000	24	16	12	6	6	7	0	**71** **(35.5%)**
	50,001– 1 lakh*	22	10	5	3	1	1	0	**42** **(21%)**
	1–1.5 lakhs	9	3	0	0	0	2	0	**14** **(7%)**
Total annual HH income slabs	1.5–2 lakhs	2	3	0	0	1	1	0	**7** **(3.5%)**
	2–2.5 lakhs	0	0	0	1	1	0	0	**2** **(1%)**
	2.5–3 lakhs	0	0	0	0	0	0	0	**0**
	3–5 lakhs	2	1	0	1	0	1	1	**6** **(3%)**
	Above 5 lakhs	1	0	0	0	0	0	0	**1** **(0.5%)**
	Total	**75** **(37.5%)**	**49** **(24.5%)**	**27** **(13.5%)**	**15** **(7.5%)**	**13** **(6.5%)**	**19** **(9.5%)**	**2** **(1%)**	**200** **(100%)**

Source: Author's field work.
Note: *One lakh is equal to 0.1 million.

the next slab of '₹25,001–50,000' (Table 4.4vi). A high percentage of those from lower income brackets are subject to HIEs on account of factors outlined earlier for NHIEs.

That HIV/AIDS has serious consequences vis-à-vis medical expenses has been confirmed by statistical tests which show *very significant* difference in total HIT expenses of the last one year pertaining to the two study samples, and this despite: (i) considering expense details of *all* members in the working age group of 18–60 years from the non-HIV/AIDS HHs as opposed to details of *only* the HIV+ respondents in case of the HIV/AIDS HHs; (ii) total annual HIT expenses of almost a quarter of the HIV/AIDS sample elements appearing to be a low and insignificant sum of 'up to ₹500' only; (iii) a relatively large number of HIV+ respondents seeking 'non-private/free' treatment from government hospitals and C&S Homes; and (iv) a few getting all expenses fully/partly reimbursed by others, unlike none in case of the non-HIV/AIDS HHs sample. That HIV/AIDS has a far adverse bearing vis-à-vis HIEs can be additionally seen by the fact that even if total HIT expenses of one year of all members of the non-HIV/AIDS HHs including those below 18 and above 60 years are included, there is still a *very significant* difference existing in the total HIT expenses of the two study samples.

4.5 Regular Monthly Medical Treatment (RMMT)

RMMT is that treatment which has to be taken on a regular basis; in the case of HIV/AIDS HHs, it includes anti-retroviral therapy (ART/ARV).

4.5.1a ART Treatment

A person living with HIV/AIDS who receives ART, that is, combination of testing, treatment and medical care can live a significantly longer and healthier life, than one who does not; treatment can even restore patients in the terminal stages of AIDS to good health, an achievement nicknamed the *Lazarus Effect* (Medhini et al. 2007a: 106). ART along with other medication, renders AIDS a chronic and treatable disease (Narain and Gilks 2004: 107). Though not a cure for AIDS, ART helps drastically reduce the *viral load* [14] and delay the onset of OIs and AIDS (Singhal and Rogers 2006: 127).

At the very outset it can be stated that RMMT expenses of HIV/AIDS HHs will be higher than that of non-HIV/AIDS HHs on account of the ART component itself which is absent in the latter. Needless to say, even if ART is free, as is the case at the government-run ART centres, it does not mean that availing the same is 100 per cent expense-free. This is because though it is free, getting the same from the centres involves expenses, the out-of-pocket expenses. Often, on account of distance, time, age and/or weak nature of the HIV+ respondents, expenses of another accompanying member cannot be discounted. Out-of-pocket expenses[15] are found to be alarmingly high in India with more than a third of the population living below the poverty line (Mehdi 2008: 8); with infected individuals often being challenged by the cost of travel, besides other associated expenses which can include loss of wage as an opportunity cost for the HIV+ person as well as for the accompanying member, if any, on account of travelling to the ART centres for getting the CD-4 and/or *viral load* count done and for receiving the 'free' ART (A. Malavia, in HRLN 2008: 152). For someone who has full blown AIDS, the out-of-pocket expenses amount to almost ₹2,000 per month, this being over and above the free treatment and medicines provided by the government, with a large number of infected people incidentally not receiving the same (ibid., 151).[16] Though not with particular reference to HIV/AIDS, but to burden of diseases in general, high out-of-pocket expenses, besides draining earnings and savings and forcing HHs into borrowings to meet the health expenditures, push HHs into debt and poverty-trap; according to an estimate 2–3 per cent people are pushed into the poverty-trap every year as a result of such expenditure (Mehdi 2008: 8).

Table 4.5.1ai highlights that majority of the HIV+ respondents at almost two-thirds the sample size were on ART, with the figures for male respondents being higher at 71.11 per cent as compared to 60.91 per cent for female respondents.[17] *No significant* association was found between taking ART and gender of the HIV+ respondent. Of those on ART, while the majority of 127 (96.9 per cent) respondents availed the free ART provided at the state ART centre, only four (3.1 per cent) took privately/market purchased ART. A total of 115 respondents on ART had to incur personal/HH

Table 4.5.1ai

Whether HIV+ respondents take ART

	No. of male resp.	Percent of male resp.	No. of female resp.	Percent of female resp.	Total	Percent of total
Yes	64	71.11	67	60.91	131	65.5
No	26	28.89	43	39.09	69	34.5
Total	90	100	110	100	200	100

Source: Author's field work.

expenses, including 111 members on free ART who had to incur out-of-pocket expenses and four who availed of market purchased ART (see Table 4.5.1aii). In case of the remaining 16 members on ART, all who were on state provided free treatment, personal out-of-pocket expenses were nil since the same were fully reimbursed/ sponsored by others.

The mean expenditure incurred on ART by all sample HHs was about ₹97 per month per HIV+ respondent. The figure becomes around ₹95 if we consider those on government ART alone, excluding those whose out-of-pocket expenses were sponsored/ reimbursed by others. The mean expenses on privately purchased ART are higher at ₹2,215 (Table 4.5.1aii).

Unlike absence of significant association between whether on ART and gender of the HIV+ respondents as mentioned earlier, there was a *significant* association between the taking of ART and gender of the HH heads, with the same being to the disadvantage of female-headed HHs. That female-headed HHs are to a disadvantage and that as referred to at the beginning that almost one-third of the sample HHs/respondents are not on ART, is a matter of concern. As field interactions revealed, it was not that the health parameters in terms of CD-4 and/or *viral load* count were always good for ART not to be taken; it was instead because the respondents did not take initiative to start or continue with the treatment on account of reasons such as high out-of-pocket expenses, long distances from the ART centre or maintaining anonymity. In Goa (and among the sample respondents themselves) as of the year 2009, many

Table 4.5.1aii

Details pertaining to ART-related monthly expenses

	N	Min (₹)	Max (₹)	Mean (₹)	SD
Total amount spent on ART by ALL sample respondents/HHs*	200	0	6,000	97.21	437.37
Total amount spent on ART by those on ART only**	131	1	6,000	148	534
Total amount spent on ART by those on government ART only***	127	1	201	83.32	52.18
Total amount spent on ART by those on ART including private ART but excluding those whose associated expenses are fully sponsored by others	115	20	6,000	169	567.20
Total amount spent by those on free government ART only (excluding those whose related expenses are fully sponsored)	111	20	201	95.19	44.63
Total amount spent by those on government ART but **excluding** those whose ART associated costs were fully sponsored; those on private. ART; and those whose other regular monthly expenses were fully sponsored^	23	20	200	104	45.29
Total amount spent by those on privately purchased ART only	4	900	6,000	2,215	2,524

Source: Author's field work.
Notes: *Including those whose expenses are fully sponsored, those without ART and those on private ART.
**Including the four on private ART and the 16 whose ART associated expenses such as transport were fully sponsored.
***Including the 16 whose related expenses were fully sponsored.
^This category represents those who are on both ART and regular monthly medicines, and who spent some money on getting both. These do not include those whose personal/HH regular monthly medical expenses are nil.

did not take ART because their CD-4 count was just above the cut-off/threshold level of 200 fixed by NACO for initiation into ART (Gautham 2008: 1; GSACS 2008: 37; Jain and Stephens 2008, 8). Under circumstances prevailing abroad or even locally in case of private treatment, these would in high probability be on ART, for in such places those with 'CD-4 < 350' are put on the same (Jain and Stephens 2008: 8–9).[18] While treatment of OIs can only alleviate suffering and extend life by a few months, access to ART helps improve life expectancy of PLWHA (Over 2004, 311), and in reducing the number of orphaned children. Statistical tests showed *no significant* association existing between whether taking ART and number of years since HIV detection.[19]

4.5.1b Other RMMT Expenses (Excluding ART)

Unlike the earlier sub-section which concerned only with the HIV/AIDS HHs, the present one is concerned with non-HIV/AIDS HHs as well. Excluding ART related expenses, 85 HIV+ respondents representing 42.5 per cent of the total HIV/AIDS sample HHs incurred 'other RMMT' expenses. The corresponding figure for the control group was less than half at 41 (20.5 per cent), despite considering details of *all* HH members irrespective of age (figures further decrease by one-third the figure at 27 if details of only those in the age group of 18–60 years are considered).[20]

The average expenses incurred by the total sample HIV/AIDS HHs on 'other RMMT' are more than twice the figure of the sample non-HIV/AIDS HHs. While the figure was ₹227 per month per HIV+ respondent, it was lower at ₹100 for non-HIV/AIDS HHs, despite the latter including expense details of *all* HH members (Table 4.5.1b). Incidentally, in case of non-HIV/AIDS HHs if details of those above 60 years are dropped, mean RMMT expenses fall to ₹55.60. If one considers only those HIV+ respondents who had to incur expenses (excluding those whose expenses were reimbursed/sponsored by others), the mean expenses were as high as ₹908 per month, as opposed to only ₹490 in case of non-HIV/AIDS HHs by *including* details of *all* members and ₹412 by *excluding* details of those over 60 years.

It needs to be noted that 'other RMMT' expenses of HIV+ respondents/HHs as shown in Table 4.5.1b are comparatively higher despite respondents often availing treatment/medicines entirely free (with nil out-of-pocket expenses): (i) on account of the

Table 4.5.1b

Comparative RMMT expenditures excluding *ART expenses*

		HIV/AIDS HHs					Non-HIV/AIDS HHs			
	N	Min (₹)	Max (₹)	Mean (₹)	SD	N	Min (₹)	Max (₹)	Mean (₹)	SD
Total amount spent by concerned HHs only	85*	.00	9,000	534	1,184	27^	60	1,500	412	378
Total amount spent by only those spending personal/HH money	50**	50	9,000	908	1,434	–	–	–	–	–
Total amount spent by those on government ART	53#	.00	4,000	363	663	–	–	–	–	–
Total amount spent by those on government ART including fully sponsored but excluding those who got their regular monthly medicines fully sponsored##	27	50	4,000	712	788	–	–	–	–	–
Total amount spent by those on government ART but excluding the four whose ART expenses were fully sponsored and those whose RMMT expenses were also fully sponsored###	23	50	4,000	782	833	–	–	–	–	–
Total amount spent by those on private ART	3	250	9,000	3,483	4,801	–	–	–	–	–
Total amount in terms of ALL sample HHs	200	.00	9,000	227	813	200^^	.00	1500	55.60	196

Source: Author's field work.

Notes: *Of these, 35 get their medical requirements free/fully sponsored. Their personal expenditures are nil.

**These exclude the 35 who were on regular monthly treatment but whose personal expenses were nil.

^These figures pertain to all HH members in the working age group of 18–60 years. If the details of those above 60 years are added, the figures will be still lower

(Table 4.5.1b Continued)

(Table 4.5.1b Continued)

than those of HIV/AIDS HHs. Including the details of the 14 (above 60 years) will provide figures as follows:- N = 41; Min. amount = ₹60; Max. amount = ₹2,000; Mean = ₹490; SD = 478

^^These figures are based as per details of all members in the age group of 18–60 years only. If the RMMT expenses of those above 60 years are alongside also considered the corresponding figures, once again lower than the ones of HIV/AIDS HHs, will be as follows:- Min. amount = .00; Max. amount = ₹2,000; Mean = ₹100; and SD = 292.

#These figures represent those who take ART as well as other RMMT. It includes 16 members who got their ART expenses fully sponsored. Incidentally 26 of these 53 members got their RMMT expenses fully sponsored as well.

##This figure excludes the 26 members whose regular monthly expenses were nil being fully sponsored by others.

###These are those who are on government ART (and who had to spend own/HH money for getting the same) as well as other RMMT.

same being obtained from government hospitals/C&S Homes/ NGOs, (ii) since they are availed at the time of regular check-up (for many this being at the time of collecting the ART doses) and (iii) on account of benefactors/NGOs bearing the out-of-pocket expense burden through reimbursement. To put things in perspective with an example, of the 44 HIV+ respondents on free government ART (who had to bear out-of-pocket expenses) and who were also on 'other RMMT', 21 got the latter at nil costs on account of afore cited reasons. However, not to diminish the impact that 'other RMMT' expenses have on HIV/AIDS HHs, it needs to be reiterated that all do not get the same free; to cite the earlier example itself, 23 respondents had to pay for the same. Incidentally, many who need 'other RMMT', either do not take the same at all, or take it on a irregular basis (time perspective) or in an improper way (dosage perspective) due to financial inadequacies.

Statistical tests showed *no significant* association between whether taking 'other RMMT' and: (i) gender of the HIV+ respondents; (ii) gender of the HH heads; and (iii) the number of years since HIV was detected. There was *no significant* association as well between whether taking 'other RMMT' and gender of the HIV+ respondents on free government ART.

4.5.2 Total RMMT Expenses

Total RMMT expenses for the HIV/AIDS respondents/HHs refer to the sum total of expenses incurred on ART (if any) and 'other RMMT'. For non-HIV/AIDS HHs, total RMMT is the same as 'other RMMT' on account of the absence of ART. Including ART related expenses to RMMT expenses makes matters only worse for HIV/AIDS HHs, despite an overwhelming number opting for the 'free' ART, on account of the associated expenses involved. Of the 131 sample respondents on ART, 56 (42.7 per cent) were on other RMMT as well.[21] Incidentally, of those on ART, 'other RMMT', or both, only 19 (9.5 per cent) respondents spent nil amount of their own since their expenses were fully sponsored/reimbursed by others (Table 4.5.2i).

Table 4.5.2ii highlights the adverse position of HIV/AIDS HHs vis-à-vis total RMMT expenses, with the average expenses of HIV+ respondents being 3.25 times the size of the control group comprising *all* members. The figure becomes worse at 5.9 times if we consider details of only those in the age group of 18–60 years (from the non-HIV/AIDS HHs sample). Similarly, pertaining to those on free ART only, excluding those whose out-of-pocket expenses were fully sponsored (whether for ART or 'other RMMT'), while

Table 4.5.2i

Summarized figures of HIV+ respondents and their RMMT including ART

	No. of respondents	Percent of total sample
Those taking ART	131	65.5
Those taking *other* RMMT	85	42.5
Those taking **only** ART but no other RMMT	75	37.5
Those taking **only** *other* RMMT but no ART	29	14.5
Those taking ART **plus** other RMMT	56	28
Those who took **neither** ART **nor** *other* RMMT	40	20
Those taking ART, RMMT, or both but spent nil amount of personal/HH money	19	9.5

Source: Author's field work.

Table 4.5.2ii

Comparative total RMMT expenditures of sample HHs

	HIV/AIDS HHs					Non-HIV/AIDS HHs				
	N	Min (₹)	Max (₹)	Mean (₹)	SD	N	Min (₹)	Max (₹)	Mean (₹)	SD
Total amount spent by those on government ART	127*	1	4,200	235	477	–	–	–	–	–
Total amount spent by those on RMMT	85**	.00	15,000	682	1746	27^	60	1,500	412	378
Total amount spent by only those spending personal/HH money	50#	60	15,000	1,112	2,182	–	–	–	–	–
Total amount spent by those on government ART but excluding those whose ART and *other* RMMT associated expenses were fully sponsored	23	150	4,200	885	856	–	–	–	–	–
Total amount spent by those on private ART	4	1,000	15,000	4,828	6,801	–	–	–	–	–
Total amount spent by ALL sample HHs	200	.00	15,000	325	1178	200^^	.00	1,500	55.60	196

Source: Author's field work.

Notes: *Including the 16 and 26 who are on fully sponsored ART and RMMT respectively.

**Including those whose actual RMMT expenses are nil.

^As was mentioned in the previous sub-section, these are figures pertaining to all HH members in the working age group of 18–60 years. If the details of those above 60 years are added as well, the figures will still be lower than those of HIV/AIDS HHs. Including the details of the 14 who were above 60 years will provide figures as follows:- N = 41; Minimum amount = ₹60; Maximum amount = ₹2,000; Mean = ₹490; and SD = 478.

^^These figures are based as per details of all members in the age group of 18–60 years only. If the RMMT expenses of those above 60 years are alongside also considered, the corresponding figures, once again lower than the ones of HIV/AIDS HHs, will be as follows:- Minimum amount = .00; Maximum amount = ₹2,000; Mean = ₹100; and SD = 292.

#These exclude those 35 who were on RMMT but whose personal expenses were nil.

the mean total RMMT expenses were ₹885/- per HIV+ respondent, it was lower at ₹490 in case of the control group, despite taking details of *all* members (figure becomes ₹412 if details of only those in the age group of 18–60 years are considered). Opting for private RMMT (including ART) can worsen matters on the expense front with the mean total RMMT expenses being a whopping ₹4,828 per HIV+ respondent.

That HIV/AIDS has a strong adverse bearing on individuals/HHs through high RMMT expenses has been unequivocally revealed by statistical test results which show *highly significant* difference in total RMMT expenses (inclusive of ART) in the two samples; and this despite considering RMMT details of *all* non-HIV/AIDS HHs members, including those above 60 years of age. Incidentally, even if the huge costs associated with ART purchased privately are ignored and instead it is assumed that the costs incurred by those on private ART was only a nominal sum of ₹95 (approximate average amount spent as out-of-pocket expenses by those incurring personal expenses on free ART),[22] the total RMMT expenses are still *very significantly* higher in HIV/AIDS HHs as compared to that of the control group.

No significant differences in RMMT expenditure exist if monthly expenses associated with ART are excluded. The absence of significant association, however, is not something to cheer about since unlike HIV/AIDS HHs where RMMT details of only the HIV+ respondents were considered, in case of the control group it was details of *all* members *irrespective* of age. That there is not much bearing can also be gauged by the fact that there was a *very significant* difference in the average RMMT expenses (*excluding* ART) when details of only those within 18–60 years are considered for the control group.

The importance of what has been mentioned vis-à-vis total RMMT expenses which are significantly high in case of HIV/AIDS HHs can be appreciated in the proper perspective if one is reminded that: (i) unlike HIV/AIDS HHs where details of *only* the HIV+ respondents were considered, in case of non-HIV/AIDS HHs it was details of *all* members; and (ii) unlike non-HIV/AIDS HHs where *all* members under RMMT had to spend own/HH money to avail of even the 'free' government treatment as out-of-pocket expenses, in case of HIV/AIDS HHs a number of respondents got their requirements free (from government hospitals/C&S Homes/ NGOs) or sponsored, with even transport costs being taken care of in the case of some.

4.6 Consolidated Viewpoint

At the HH level one apparent impact of HIV/AIDS is the increased spending on treatment and care of infected members. As UNESC/ESCAP (2004: 4) brings out, HIV/AIDS affects poor HHs disproportionately, with poor PLWHA who have no access to treatment becoming susceptible faster to OIs and losing their ability to engage in remunerative work. Incidentally, while in case of those who can afford treatment, the prohibitive costs can lead to the diversion of finances from other essential areas, thereby enforcing a cycle of impoverishment; poor diagnosis/ prognosis combined with insufficient information on treatment of AIDS or OIs can result in wasteful expenditure on ineffective health care (ibid.).

Related to the issue of poverty, HIV/AIDS is a contributor of *iatrogenic poverty*, that is, poverty induced by medicine, which occurs when in order to access medicine, the entire family becomes impoverished (A. Malavia, in HRLN 2008: 152). This is of particular concern in India where medical treatment is supposedly provided free by the government in public hospitals. Poverty can be a fallout despite the same since it is the often the district hospitals that are the centres of all treatment services including ART, with PLWHA often being challenged by the travel and other out-of-pocket expenses (ibid.). According to F. Khan (HRLN 2008: 156) though ART is free, 30–40 per cent of the money which a HIV+ person has is spent on making hospital trips and for buying medicines, with not much remaining for other needs including food. To make matters worse an HIV+ person on account of taking leave for testing or treatment, gets reduced salary, with occasions being there where only half month salary is earned (ibid.).

Unlike earlier sections which dealt with particular medical aspects such as NHIEs, HIEs and RMMT, the present section attempts at providing a consolidated perspective,[23] albeit with a caveat that this approach is fraught with a few weaknesses and limitations (despite the same it has been nevertheless adopted with the aim of discussing the issue from a relatively un-researched and un-documented perspective; one which will provide not only a *broad indication* of the harsh realities facing HIV/AIDS HHs, but that which will also provoke a broader debate and even further research). Considering the average total annual HH medical expenses of HIV/AIDS HHs which were ₹12,991 per HH (see Chapter 3), and figures obtained in earlier sections for RMMT, NHIT and HIT, it can be said that while average RMMT expenses of HIV+ respondents alone for one year constitutes about 30 per cent of the total annual HH medical expenditure, the share of annual HIT expenses constitutes approximately another 32 per cent. Pertaining to NHIEs, assuming there were no other illness episodes during the year other than those taking place in the last one month,[24] the share of expenses get to be about 9 per cent of the total annual HH medical expenditure. From the above it can be seen that the total annual medical expenses of the HIV+ respondents themselves is a minimum of ₹9,235 per person, constituting about 71 per cent of the total annual HH medical expenses. The balance of ₹3,756 approximately goes to cover: (i) NHIT expenses, if any, of earlier months; and/or (ii) medical expenses of other HH members.

The grave situation faced by HIV+ respondents can be understood better by seeing the corresponding figure for non-HIV/AIDS HHs (average total HH annual medical expenses ₹2,555) wherein, despite taking into account details of *all* members (18–60 years), the figure of total medical expenses was only ₹1,309 per HH. Unlike the high percentage share of total annual medical expenses of HIV+ respondents to the total annual HH medical expenses standing at a *minimum* of about 71 per cent, the figure was only about 51 per cent for the control group.[25]

On account of non-consideration of NHIT details of earlier months, the cited figures pertaining to total annual medical expenses of the HIV+ respondents are only approximate in nature. If the sum of ₹9,235 is considered as approximate *minimum* average 'total annual medical expense' per HIV+ respondent, the per capita annual total medical expenses for *other* HIV/AIDS HH members will be about ₹1,356 per annum.[26] If we assume that figures pertaining to total annual medical expenses of the HIV+ respondents and other HH members as cited are a true approximation, medical expenses of the former will be at least 6.8 times the figure of other members. Interestingly, though the figure for other HIV/AIDS HH members is far less than the figure for HIV+ respondents, it is nevertheless relatively higher than the per capita figures for non-HIV/AIDS HHs which was approximately ₹570 per HH member per annum, and this despite more members going for private treatment and with none getting their treatment related expenses reimbursed/sponsored by others. The higher figures of medical expenses for other HH members in HIV/AIDS HHs is partly on account of the fact that there are other HIV+ members living alongside (in the present study, excluding the sample respondents, there were additional 104 PLWHA in the sample HHs). Incidentally, a substantial part of the said expenses of HIV/AIDS HHs will be a part of the unknown earlier NHIT expenses of the sample HIV+ respondents themselves.

The total medical expenses of the HIV+ respondents considered at ₹9,235 per person (under the bold assumption), is a figure equal to at least 14.63 per cent in terms of 'total annual HH income' (only 1.22 per cent in case of the control group comprising *all* members within 18–60 years), with the figure being 15.91 per cent in terms of the total annual wage income (1.26 per cent for the control group). Alternatively, instead of considering the total medical expenses of the HIV+ respondents on a *per annum* basis, if we take expenses on *per last month* basis and relate the same to the average total HH income per month, the percentage of the former to the latter becomes more than one-third at 35 per cent in case of HIV+ respondents (only 2.45 per cent in case of the control group). Findings of the present study have been affirmed by other studies. Ramamurthy (2004: 234), indicated that HIV+ individuals on an average spend between 10 and 30 per cent of their annual incomes on HIV related health expenditures, with most of the expenses being on medicines; with the impact being more on lower income groups besides those who had dependants. According to Gupta (1998), 10–30 per cent of the annual income of an individual may be spent on treatment (in Kadiyala and Barnett 2004: 1891).

Total annual HH medical expenses as a percentage of 'total annual HH income' and total annual HH wage income is 20.58 per cent and 22.39 per cent respectively (corresponding figures for non-HIV/AIDS HHs were as low as 2.38 and 2.45 per cent respectively). If not for the total annual medical expenses of the HIV+ respondents, the medical expenses of HIV/AIDS HHs would have been less by at least 71 per cent. Likewise, if not for the mean total annual medical expenses of the HIV+ respondents standing at ₹9,235 approximately, the average total 'other annual HH consumption expenditure' would have been reduced by 25.27 per cent, enabling HHs to save more and/or spend on non-medical HH requirements including food, which are otherwise sacrificed. In contrast to the high figure for the HIV/AIDS HHs sample, the corresponding figure for non-HIV/AIDS HHs sample despite taking *all* members (18–60 years) was only 4.79 per cent. The total annual medical expenditure of the HIV+ respondents forms a minimum of about 10.5 per cent of the 'total annual HH consumption expenditure' (inclusive of food, regular monthly HH expenditures and other annual HH consumption expenditures; and excluding remittances and savings/investments). The corresponding figure for non-HIV/AIDS HHs despite details of *all* (18–60 years) is only 1.53 per cent. The average total annual medical expenses of the HIV+ respondents themselves would have sufficed to take care of total food expenses of at least 3.5 months of the total sample HIV/AIDS HHs. Incidentally, while size of the total annual HH medical expenditures to 'total annual HH consumption expenditures' (as per the above mentioned definition) was equal to about 14.82 per cent, the size of the total annual HH medical expenditure to 'other annual HH consumption expenditure' was equal to 35.57 per cent. The corresponding figures for non-HIV/AIDS HHs were only 2.98 and 9.36 per cent respectively.

In fine, to portray the gravity of HIV/AIDS on health, if not for the total annual medical expenses incurred on the HIV+ respondents,

HIV/AIDS HHs would have been able to: (i) reduce 'total annual HH consumption expenditure'; (ii) increase consumption of non-medical items including food, clothing/footwear, durable goods and entertainment; (iii) increase savings/investments; (iv) reduce borrowings and associated remittances; and/or (v) decrease dissavings and dependence on UUI. Incidentally, the total annual medical expenses of just one person per HH, that is, the HIV+ respondent, who often: (a) avails free government/NGO/C&S Homes treatment; (b) benefits from partly/fully sponsored treatment; and/or (c) does not take treatment due to financial problems, are greater than the average dissavings amounting to ₹8,771 of HIV/AIDS HHs of the last one year (see Chapter 3). From the point of view of losses incurred, things can only worsen particularly for HHs from the lower income brackets if loss of income due to absenteeism from work of self or caregiver is also factored in. Additionally, it needs to be remembered that losses arising to HIV/AIDS HHs will be high not only because of the high medical expenses, but also because of a loss of earning capacities/ employment, especially if we consider the 'young' average age (mid-thirties) and age groups that majority of the HIV+ respondents belong(ed) to (see Section 4.2 and *Appendix I:* Table AI.x). Leaving aside the sample respondents, the vast majority of PLWHA belong to the economically productive age groups, with 30 per cent of the infected in India being in the age group of 15–29 years itself;[27] with 40 per cent of all new HIV infections being among those in the age group of 15–24 years.[28] Losses can only compound if there are multiple HIV+ HH members and if those getting support from external agencies stop getting the same.

Giving proper and timely treatment though entails huge expenses even leading to *iatrogenic poverty* is nevertheless of utmost necessity. Not only does it provide relief, prolong life and productive years, improve well being, delay onset of OIs and AIDS, increase life-expectancy and decrease number of orphans,[29] it also raises lifetime HH income and improves parental care (Bell et al. 2004: 124). Studies such as Bloom et al. (2000; 2004) show a rise in output, labour productivity and/or per capita income through improved life-expectancy (in ADB 2004: 45). It is claimed that with medical care and nutritional management, an HIV+ person can live a reasonably long and healthy life (Gautham 2008: 1). To put in perspective the importance of food and nutrition itself in the well-being of PLWHA, it has been claimed that of those who were able to access ART, the ones malnourished when they started the treatment were six times more likely to die than those not malnourished (A. Malavia, in HRLN 2008: 151–152).

4.7 Miscellaneous

4.7.1 Private Treatment

The treatment for HIV infection with allopathic medicines is said to run to even over ₹2,00,000 per annum, a sum which most Indians can ill afford, with the treatment to be taken till death (Ramaiah 2008: 65). Around a decade back it was found that depending on the combination of drugs, a year's supply could range from ₹42,000 to ₹1,20,000 with only about one to 2 per cent of the infected people in the country being able to afford drugs at such prices (Sengupta 2000: 124). On account of prohibitive costs for private treatment, with treatment needed to be taken without break over an indefinite period of time, for any medical exigency there are generally more HIV/AIDS HHs which depend on free government treatment than the paid private treatment that non-HIV/AIDS HHs usually rely upon; a reliance of the latter HHs on private treatment due to affordability, less frequency of illness episodes, convenience and supposedly prompt and good quality treatment. If one takes an overview of the source of annual medical treatment, primary dependence of sample HIV+ respondents during the last one year was:- (i) government treatment: 27 per cent; (ii) private treatment: 6.5 per cent; (iii) both government and private treatment: 18 per cent; and (iv) government and NGOs/C&S Homes treatment: 48.5 per cent. Of the 54 HIV+ respondents availing government treatment, nine (4.5 per cent of the total sample) used to take only private treatment earlier but had to totally switch over due to financial difficulties.

Related to private HIV/AIDS treatment, it is often the treatment that is preferred, at least in the beginning on account of keeping ones identity and HIV+ status under wraps, and possibly, as the Commission on Macroeconomics and Health (CMH) found in 2000–2001, due to the deficiency of the public sector in India towards health care, as 5/6th of all health related spending which occur in the private sector is a possible indicator of (Sachs 2008: 4).[30] Though only a few sample respondents were currently on private treatment, there were nevertheless others who were partly or exclusively on the same earlier before switching to government/NGO provided treatment (see also Pandey 2006: 12). Field interactions revealed, at least in the context of the socio-economic categories of HHs under study, over-dependence on private treatment for ART or 'other RMMT' itself, has often led to two adverse outcomes both having serious economic ramifications:

1. Households gradually wipe out their savings/investments/ assets on expensive treatment with hardly any assets remaining for future needs. Matters get compounded because alongside earning capacities too drop gradually, with present consumption of non-medical goods including food often getting compromised upon. The prohibitive private medical costs that cannot be sustained always by all for a long and indefinite period of time can be put in perspective with a glance at the pricing of drugs, where leaving aside surgical procedures, ART treatment itself can cost between ₹1,300 and 3,900 per month for the *first-line* treatment; about ₹8,300 per month for the *second-line* treatment; and a whopping ₹80,000–1,00,000 per month for a more superior, often called the *third-line* treatment;[31] and

2. ART is a lifelong commitment (Jain and Stephens 2008: 9). Adherence, taking the drugs exactly as prescribed: on time and in accordance with any diet/lifestyle restrictions and for the person's lifetime, is a must in case of HIV/AIDS (ibid.). Failure to take doses properly can be very harmful and can have the following fallouts: (i) failure of drug to suppress HIV; (ii) development of drug resistance; (iii) drugs not being

absorbed properly by the body and hence getting wasted; (iv) virus not getting suppressed and hence there being no benefit to the individual; and (v) person taking the drugs still having to bear the severe negative side effects (Jain and Stephens 2008: 9). At least over 90–95 per cent adherence levels are required; missing on the drug cannot be more than one dose a month (ibid.; Medhini et al. 2007a: 108). Dependence on private treatment, especially considering the socio-economic background of the HHs, has often contributed to respondents being unable to spend on a regular basis and on the right dosages of medicines. Medicines are often skipped or dosages reduced contrary to medical advice. This can and has caused irreversible damage to the health status of HIV+ respondents, with not only health deteriorating further, but also a need arising to put them on stronger and higher dosages of drugs, or changing the line of treatment itself, all entailing higher expenses. It needs to be noted that with the best combination of drugs itself, infections keep spreading with HIV developing multi-drug resistance,[32] thereby making treatment harder (Israni 2001: 191–192).[33] Not taking proper treatment makes matters worse. This is not to say that it is only privately purchased treatment that is likely to cause drop in adherence levels. Even with government/NACO provided ART, a poor adherence has been recorded due to factors such as time involved at ART centres, breakdown of CD-4 (GSACS 2008: vii) and *viral load* count machines, long distances to ART centres, lack of total privacy, etc. (see also C. Gonsalves, in HRLN 2008: 41–48). Studies indicate that more than half of those who were fortunate to start with the treatment[34] were not adhering to their treatment regimen by the end of the first year itself due to the high costs of drugs and tests (Stephens and Jain 2008: 19). However, leaving aside the limitations of free treatment, adherence can get worse with private treatment due to prohibitive costs itself. As field observations revealed many HIV+ people on private treatment, on knowing of their incapacity to sustain the treatment, either die due to discontinuation, or switch over to treatment provided by government hospitals/NGOs/C&S Homes,[35] which quite often is a little too late (see also Pandey 2006: 12).

4.7.2 Discrimination

Discrimination, which includes health/medical care related discrimination, only fuels the fire of economic disasters faced by HIV/AIDS individuals/HHs. Discrimination can be: *financial incapacity to pay* related (on account of poor background of HHs in general) and *sickness/stigma* related. While private health care service providers being 'for profit' enterprises cannot guarantee equity of care especially to those 'bad clients' with chronic diseases, pre-existing medical conditions and those who cannot make payments on a regular basis (Krishnamoorthy 2009: 9); government health facilities too are often culprits at the time of dispensing treatment especially in case of PLWHA (see also Nagarajan 2007: 7). Let alone HIV/AIDS, state-run health care services/schemes that are meant for all, rarely reach those in need and often require influence to be accessible; patients have inevitably to purchase medicines from the market though they are supposedly available free in government hospitals (Nair 2009b: 2), thus (in)directly contributing towards additional economic burden. Common examples of fallouts faced by sample HIV+ respondents on account of medical discrimination[36] include: (i) further treatment is stopped forthright; (ii) improper, medically unsound and dangerous home remedy is adopted;[37] and (iii) there is delay in seeking treatment, which worsens the ailment and raises the cost of treatment on account of further deterioration in health. Leaving aside the numerous non-economic fallouts that are bound to arise, all the above contribute to fall in earning capacities due to poor employability, with a few even becoming permanently unemployable as well due to irreversible damage to health.[38]

4.7.3 Others

The situation on the treatment front for HIV/AIDS HHs can be worse than what has already been highlighted, if they have other sick members, particularly HIV+ members. The medical expenses of these latter members even if not high at present, can go up in subsequent years due to gradual progression through the stages of HIV infection. On account of financial difficulties caused by HIV/AIDS, often HIV-negative members as well do not get timely and proper treatment for their ailments. In contrast, non-HIV/AIDS HHs, as mentioned earlier, are better placed vis-à-vis treatment despite: (i) considering details of *all* HH members (18–60 years); (ii) more going for 'paid' private treatment; and (iii) none getting medical expenses fully reimbursed/sponsored by others, unlike their HIV/AIDS counterparts.

To take care of rising expenses and falling income HIV/AIDS HHs often adopt a variety of coping mechanisms, a number of which were mentioned in the earlier chapters, such as, wife, minor children and those above 60 years taking up remunerative employment; taking assistance from NGOs; resorting to borrowings from relatives/friends, employers, financial institutions and money-lenders; resorting to dissavings; and depending on UUI. The present study has revealed that besides the above, other coping mechanisms made use of by sample HHs include: availing support from extended family[39] and mortgaging assets. While 46.5 per cent sample respondents availed of the former, 12.5 per cent made use of the latter. The coping mechanisms are either absent, or play only an insignificant role in case of non-HIV/AIDS HHs, where the majority manage needs with own resources, comprising present earnings and/or past savings.

Notes

1. The same are important to understand the economic impact of AIDS, the key attributes of which are large number of cases, costly treatment and mortality that is concentrated among working-age adults.

2. Similar patterns are observed even if extreme sample elements from the higher end are ignored.
3. With reference to NHIEs in the present study, while *frequently* refers to a member being ill four to five times a month or more; *continuously* refers to a member being regularly ill (i.e. every single or alternate day).
4. Majority of these did not seek treatment despite being frequently or continuously ill. Incidentally, all these belonged to HHs having a low total annual HH income. While 10 (33.3 per cent) belonged to the 'up to ₹25,000' per annum category, 13 (43.3 per cent) belonged to the '₹25,001–50,000' bracket, with the remaining six (20 per cent) and one (3.3 per cent) belonging to the '₹50,001–1,00,000' and '₹1,00,001–1,50,000' brackets respectively.
5. It was not financial inadequacies, which was a primary reason among those whose HIV+ status was detected over a relatively longer period.
6. WHO classifies the HIV infection into four clinical stages based on the infections and the performance scale (Pradhan et al. 2006: 116–117).
7. OIs are those caused by otherwise harmless microorganisms that can become pathogenic when the host's resistance is impaired (WCC 2002: 110). While OIs decrease the CD-4 count, thereby weakening the HIV+ individual further; poor CD-4 count, in turn, can make the HIV+ person vulnerable to more OIs.
8. While the mean age of total HIV+ sample respondents was 36.50 years (SD: 8.73); the mean age of those sick last month but not continuously/frequently (43 in number) was 35.12 years (SD: 7.87).
9. Fourteen were sick *frequently* and eight *continuously*.
10. Or 23 per cent if one considers the entire sample.
11. Liquidation of assets and/or borrowings has also been reported by other studies as well including Pradhan et al. (2006).
12. That the mean number of days hospitalized is high in case of HIV+ respondents can be better appreciated by seeing that even if couple of extreme sample elements are *trimmed*, average number of days hospitalized is still considerably higher at 24.72 (SD: 23.58).
13. Reimbursement or sponsoring of expenses which is done at times by NGOs or benefactors in case of HIV+ respondents, does not usually happen in case of non-HIV/AIDS HHs. While HIV+ respondents who got their medical expenses including out-of-pocket expenses fully reimbursed by others were not considered for deriving the mean values pertaining to expenses as mentioned herein; of those respondents considered, some got additional amounts over and above their own, provided by others.
14. An untreated HIV+ person has thousands or even millions of HIV particles in every millilitre of blood. This is known as the *viral load*. Lower the *viral load*, better it is for the recovery of the immune system. The aim of ART is to suppress the level of HIV in the body to a very low level, ideally below 50 *copies* of HIV per millilitre (50/mm³) of blood (Jain and Stephens 2008: 5).
15. According to WHO, those payments made by the patient at the point of receiving health care; with the definition taking a cross sectional view of the point of interface between the patient and the service provider (A. Malavia, in HRLN 2008: 152).
16. In the recent past, despite much initiative, experience, spending and global funding, 2.6 lakh (i.e. 0.26 million) PLWHA in India were still in dire need of ART (Sinha 2010b: 11).

17. Incidentally, of those not on ART, many were on urgent need of the same, but were not availing primarily due to extreme financial constraints and lack of support. This, besides putting life to greater vulnerability, was also reducing the productive life or the respondents.
18. See also AIDS.org: http://www.aids.org/factsheets/124-t-cell-tests.html, accessed July 2010.
19. The need of being on ART is not dependent *per se* on the number of years since contracting HIV; it depends on circumstances such as general pre-disposition, CD-4 count, *viral load* count, etc., which in turn are often influenced by factors such as nutritional status, OIs, etc.
20. Pertaining to non-HIV/AIDS HHs, while about two-thirds at 65.9 per cent (27 respondents) belonged to the 18–60 years age bracket, 34.1 per cent (14 respondents) represented those above 60 years (in one case vis-à-vis the latter details pertained to two members of the same HH).
21. While 53 (41.7 per cent) out of 127 on 'free' ART were also on 'other RMMT', figures were three (75 per cent) out of four with regard to those on private ART. This is in lieu of the mean ₹2,215 spent by those on private ART (see Table 4.5.1aii).
22. This is in lieu of the mean ₹2,215 spent by those on private ART (see Table 4.5.1aii).
23. Pertaining to the sample HIV/AIDS HHs, during the course of last one year alone, 50 per cent HIV+ respondents were subject to all three: NHIEs, HIEs and RMMT, irrespective of whether treatment was availed; whether the persons suffered NHIEs during the last one month or earlier; and whether the treatment was free/fully sponsored. Of the remaining, while 67 (33.5 per cent) respondents were subject to least two of the mentioned three during the year, 26 (13 per cent) were subject to at least one. Only seven (3.5 per cent) respondents were free of all three. Interestingly, with regard to those 'illness free' during the last one year, either some were exposed to HIV related illness (and treatment) in the past (entailing expenses extending to as high as even over ₹3,00,000), or, in the concerned HHs some other HIV+ member, not part of the present study, were currently undergoing treatment.
24. This bold assumption, though not in consonance with ground reality since there were illness episodes in earlier months as well, was made for the purpose of arriving at *minimum* average NHIE expenditure figures per HIV+ respondent. Details of earlier months are unavailable since the objective of the study was primarily to analyse NHIT expense details of the last one month only; an objective similar to the NCAER/UNDP/NACO study (Pradhan et al. 2006). Needless to say, it is not easy to get respondents to provide minute details pertaining to NHIEs of the entire year due to the large number of illness episodes experienced in general, with treatment often not taken for certain episodes, with some episodes getting only home remedy. On account of numerous complexities involved, primarily on account of the very nature of the study, there is no full-proof method, post-data collection, of finding/estimating the correct NHIE expense figures for the earlier 11 months, only on the basis of knowing the number of illness episodes that took place earlier and expense figures of the last month. This is due to reasons such as, treatment costs are not always the same; treatment is not always taken; even if/when taken, treatment does not always involve personal costs (expenses get reimbursed occasionally by others like relations, benefactors and NGOs);

the nature of earlier illness episode(s) may be different to that/those of the last month; source of treatment may be different in different months, etc. Considering the nature of the assumption, the percentage share of medical expenses of the HIV+ respondents to the total annual HH medical expenses could only get higher than that cited herein.

25. The balance expenditure was primarily incurred on those '<18 and > 60 years', though a small part would still be on those within 18–60 years, since NHIEs of the earlier months were not considered.

26. Average of 2.77 members per HH, excluding the HIV+ respondent (see *Appendix I*: Table AI.v).

27. See 'HIV highest in 15 to 29 age group'. *TOI*, Goa, 2 June 2008, 7.

28. See 'Youth form 40% of HIV patients'. *TOI*, Goa, 25 June 2008, 3.

29. HIV is notorious for the creation of a large population of child-headed HHs and orphans by taking away lives of parents through AIDS (see Verma et al. 2002, in Medhini et al. 2007b: 1090). In addition to suffering from emotional deficiencies, these orphans are often subjected to food insecurity and malnourishment (Medhini et al. 2007b: 1090); besides insufficient education (Ainsworth and Filmer 2002; Case et al. 2004, Evans and Miguel 2004, Yamano and Jayne 2004, all in Werker et al. 2007: 18), all precursors for a bleak and uncertain future. Incidentally, girls orphaned by AIDS additionally face 'property grabbing' when their parents die, leaving them with no means of support (Medhini et al. 2007a: 456).

30. Public health expenditure in India as a proportion of total health expenditure is only 16 per cent; much less than in Ethiopia, Nigeria and Pakistan where it is 36, 28 and 23 per cent respectively (Ramachandran and Rajalakshmi 2009: 25).

31. Market prices in approximate figures of commonly prescribed drugs as per recommended dosages have been provided as factual examples of the prohibitive costs of treatment especially for an average Indian: *First-line* treatment (four common options)—(i) TRIOMUNE-30 tabs: ₹1,324 per month; (ii) DUOVIR-N tabs: ₹1,544 per month; (iii) VIRADAY tabs: ₹3,900 per month; (iv) generic combination of Zidovudine, Lamivudine and Efavirenz: ₹3,200 per month. *Second-line* treatment—LOPIMUNE, TENVIR-EM and Zidovudine: ₹8,316 per month. *Third-line* treatment—Fusion inhibitors: ₹80,000–1,00,000 per month. Incidentally, while the treatment course prescribed depends on various parameters of the patient; each has its own side effects (see Ramaiah 2008: 67–74). Often additional treatment is recommended alongside on a regular basis. Despite, or on account of its prohibitive price, the *third-line* treatment is often not available in the market.

32. One HIV virus can make 10 billion copies of itself in a day, with a mutation rate of one in 10,000 (Gaitonde 2001, in Singhal and Rogers 2006: 46–47).

33. To cite a related example of TB which is often associated with HIV/AIDS in order to see the economic dimension of the fallout of getting infected with drug resistant versions of illnesses: while normal TB can be treated in six months, drug resistant TB takes over two years, with drugs being less potent and more toxic; while standard TB drugs cost US$20, drug resistant TB medicines cost up to US$5,000 (Sinha 2010c: 11).

34. At the turn of the century only about 2.2 per cent of PLWHA in India were receiving ART.

35. The switching is dangerous because often private practitioners put PLWHA on ART once CD-4 count becomes '<350'. However, if one switches to government ART, one gets it only if the CD-4 count is '≤200'. Hence, if at the time of switching if ones CD-4 count was '>200', one does not get the free ART. This is dangerous since once started, ART cannot be stopped. PLWHA often and consciously, despite high risk involved, decrease their CD-4 count to '<200' for availing the free ART.

36. Medical discrimination is faced by PLWHA even in present times in state-run public health services despite Government of India memorandum No. 11020/29/1198/NACCO (Admn ART) dated 26 August 2008, with directives for compliance of the Supreme Court to ensure the rights of PLHA.

37. In one case, on account of denial of treatment despite being kept in/near the operation theatre for the entire day ostensibly for treatment, an HIV+ individual resorted to self removal of the ulcer/abscess at home which in reality necessitated a surgical procedure to be performed by a medical practitioner under local anesthesia and necessitating hospital stay.

38. In one case, delay in providing timely treatment led to a HIV+ person becoming permanently blind; costly treatment in the range of ₹80,000–1,00,000 provided by the state subsequently was not sufficient to reverse the damage already caused.

39. Relations not directly part of the HH; with regard to HIV/AIDS HHs these relations are usually from the wife's side (64 per cent of the cases).

5

The Way Ahead

HIV/AIDS is like a huge rock in society. Only if everyone in society keeps breaking the rock into smaller pieces will it eventually become dust (Sommai Punnyakamo 2001, in Singhal and Rogers 2006: 242).

5.1 The Present...A Summary

At the very outset two things need to be affirmed in the context of the present study: (i) though the findings/inferences are primarily with reference to sample respondents/HHs on account of the sampling techniques and statistical tools used, nevertheless, conclusions drawn are very much indicative and reflective of the ground situation for other HIV/AIDS HHs as well, especially for those from the lower income brackets; and (ii) the findings though reiterating unambiguously the serious nature of economic fallouts of HIV/AIDS and the urgent need for corrective action, it does not do so to imply that HIV/AIDS is the only infection/illness that needs to be addressed urgently or at the cost of other illnesses—other ailments/diseases not part of the present study could be serious as well in their own ways with regard to their economic fallouts.[1]

The present study has indisputably highlighted the severe nature of economic hardships HIV/AIDS spews on individuals and HHs. The same is reflective not only via a large number of HHs involved vis-à-vis the fallouts faced, but also in terms of adverse mean values involved. Adversities faced by HIV/AIDS

HHs/individuals are not only higher than those of their matched non-HIV/AIDS counterparts, but also the same are in fact often *very significantly* higher. HIV/AIDS has made HHs poorer; severely challenging even the basic living conditions.

Gender plays a biased role on many occasions vis-à-vis HIV/AIDS contributed economic fallouts, with female-headed HHs and/or female HIV+ respondents facing significantly more adverse conditions and hardships than their male counterparts. The absence of significant gender based hardships or the presence of gender-neutral nature of impacts (unlike more biases against females in non-HIV/AIDS HHs), whenever it is so, is not a reflection of better conditions for females; it only reflects that adversities are bad for all irrespective of gender and that females have reduced some of the differences, despite their significantly adverse position in terms of total annual HH income, through adoption of numerous coping mechanisms, each having their own burden and undesirability.

The study has shown that HIV/AIDS has serious adverse impact on *income* and *employment*. While both fall due to reasons such as increased absenteeism, episodes of sickness, changes in jobs and caregiving duties; death of an earning AIDS member makes matters worse, with the income source getting permanently discontinued. With regard to *health* and *medical expenditure*, while the former keeps deteriorating in terms of the number of respondents/HHs facing illness episodes and the number of illness episodes faced each year; the latter which is extremely high, makes HH income/savings dwindle, forcing HHs to cut essential non-medical consumption, besides making HHs depend much on dissavings, borrowings and/or UUI. Incidentally, the medical expenses of HIV+ respondents are higher than the medical expenses of *all* HHs members of non-HIV/AIDS taken together; that too, in spite of 'free' medical treatment dispensed by the government (and particularly availed of by HIV/AIDS individuals/HHs).

HIV/AIDS greatly influences the *annual HH income* and *expenditure flows*. With regard to the latter, barring extremely high medical expenses, the consumption expenses of HIV/AIDS HHs in general are smaller than those of their counterparts. Additionally, while savings and investments are hardly worth the mention in

HIV/AIDS HHs, remittances are comparatively high, a reflection of greater borrowings. Food insufficiency is experienced by HIV/AIDS HHs despite much dependence on partly/fully sponsored food, dependence without which the survival of HHs itself would have been under threat. The serious impact that HIV/AIDS has can also be seen through a glance of HH income inflows. While total annual HH income plays a major role in case of non-HIV/AIDS HHs, in case of HIV/AIDS HHs it is borrowings and UUI.

Economic impacts of HIV/AIDS can only get worse than that recorded in the study if among others: (i) external assistance is not considered and/or the same gets reduced/stopped in the future; (ii) fall in the present education levels and asset holdings due to HIV/AIDS affects future earnings/economic conditions; (iii) there are two or more HIV+ members in the HH; (iv) those currently sick are unable to take up remunerative employment again; (v) repayment of borrowed amounts accumulating over the years becomes a problem especially considering additional loss of income/employment and diminishing asset holdings, and with amount raised through UUI being uncertain because of their very nature; and (vi) the steep rise in food inflation running into double digits experienced post-survey is additionally considered (see Shrinivasan 2010: 13). The economic dilemmas for HHs get compounded on account of perceived, potential and/or actual discrimination of different types facing HIV+ respondents.

In fine, among others, the three major and unique findings of the present study (findings either unrecorded or not easily available in the existing literature; yet those reflecting the severe nature of the economic crises facing individuals/HHs) are as follows: (i) to make up for shortfall in HH income and meet HH requirements, there is high dependence on the part of HIV/AIDS HHs on partly/fully sponsored food, especially among female-headed HHs; (ii) to meet HH expenses including medical and to cover deficits, besides relying much on borrowings, there is significantly high dependence on UUI (particularly among female-headed HHs); and (iii) the total annual medical expenses of the HIV+ respondents alone (despite treatment being primarily availed at 'free' public health centres, treatment being partly/fully sponsored, or treatment even not availed at all due to financial constraints) is significantly greater than the total annual medical expenditure of *all* members of non-HIV/AIDS HH taken together. Incidentally, pertaining to income/employment, the high toll HIV/AIDS bears on affected HHs forces many to adopt coping mechanisms including unwanted ones such as minor children and those above 60 years of age taking up remunerative employment, or HIV+ members themselves taking up additional employment; all options which are generally conspicuous by their absence in non-HIV/AIDS HHs, even in the eventuality of loss of income/employment.

5.2 The Future...The Way Ahead

The study has revealed numerous multi-faceted adverse economic fallouts of HIV/AIDS on individuals and HHs. The economic impact of HIV/AIDS for India, with a huge population of over a billion and a work force of 400 million (about 92 per cent in the unorganized sector) can be overwhelming; for such a labour force in the unorganized sector, there is only a thin line (or even no lines) separating the work and living place (CEC 2004). While the present scenario for HIV/AIDS HHs is bad due to high medical expenses and a fall in income and consumption levels; the future too is anything but promising on account of current decline in education, savings and assets, besides the high-debt burden. Alleviation of the adverse fallouts thus assumes great importance.

The choice of any appropriate intervention, for government or 'others' (such as NGOs) particularly in developing countries has to be on the basis of cost-effectiveness (Gupta and Panda 2002: 190). Besides a societal perspective, cost-effectiveness necessitates focus on issues such as indirect benefits to those affected and others, with there being a need to attain a net gain instead of only replacement in efforts (World Bank 1997, in Gupta and Panda 2002: 190). It has been accepted that involvement of 'others' besides partnerships with the government are critical in the context of cost-effectiveness on the basis of comparative advantage, compensation for lack of skills and saving of resources (ibid.).

Implementation of alleviatory and preventive measures with regard to HIV/AIDS is an arduous and challenging task, particularly in the context of developing countries. While scarcity of resources,[2] illiteracy and the absence of quick decision making in general are serious impediments; strong stigma itself comes in the way of seeking proper solutions vis-à-vis HIV/AIDS. Notwithstanding the important role that 'others' such as NGOs can play along with the government vis-à-vis alleviation in the context of HIV/AIDS, the dominating role that the latter has to bear comes into prime focus on account of the market failures that exist vis-à-vis HIV prevention (Israni 2001; see also Drummond and Kelly 2006); market failures which at least in the initial stages, the government is apparently in the position to handle appropriately.[3]

Recommendations or measures towards alleviation vis-à-vis the present study have been provided in two broad parts: preventive[4] and 'curative'. The latter, meant for a post-infection scenario, includes those directly related in tackling HIV as a medical condition[5] and those related to 'curing' the adverse economic fallouts of HIV/AIDS on individuals/HHs. Incidentally, some measures are both preventive and curative in nature.[6]

5.2.1 Preventive Measures

The best way of taking care of the adverse impact of HIV/AIDS is to *prevent* people from contracting the infection itself. Vast literature points towards advocacy, effectiveness and long-run profitability of preventive measures, over post HIV contracted 'curative' measures. While according to Rao (2000a: 55), one certainty with regard to the rising costs of the HIV epidemic in Asia is that investment in prevention to reduce the spread of HIV and its costs to society is a major economy in comparison to the cost of damage control at a later stage which will grow exponentially; according to World Bank reports, US$1 invested in prevention is equal to about US$67 saved on care and support (HRLN 2008: 34). ADB (2004: viii) also shows that spending on HIV prevention and AIDS care is justified by the high economic returns that can be expected to flow from such spending. Schoub (1995: 213) reiterates that with ethical dilemmas in the developing world already suffering from other diseases, malnutrition and inadequate facilities, there is greater priority for preventive health programmes, including AIDS, as compared to treatment costs. The Report of the National Commission on Macroeconomics and Health (2005) on a related aspect highlights that prevention of diseases is the most cost-effective strategy for a country facing scarce resources (in Mehdi 2008: 8). The maintenance of health involves not only the treatment of the disease but also the prevention of the disease, with the latter potentially achievable via social-environmental change rather than only direct medical services (McGuire et al. 1997: 2 and 14). Even the possible arrival of a safe, effective and affordable vaccine for HIV is not to be considered as a replacement for other HIV prevention strategies, but instead it is to be delivered as part of a comprehensive HIV prevention programme inclusive of other behavioural and health promotion interventions (Esparza and Osmanov 2004: 349–350).

The importance of education in general and in the context of HIV/AIDS prevention in particular, cannot be diminished in any way (see also Albert and Williams 1998: 96). With around three new HIV cases being detected in Goa each day at the ICTCs[7] itself and with the sexual route accounting for even as high as 94–96 per cent of new infections even at present, it is obvious that ignorance of preventive measures through appropriate behavioural changes have not taken place. While various studies (see Nair 2009c: 4) and reports such as Behavioural Surveillance Survey (GSACS 2005–2006: 47) and NFHS-3[8] have highlighted insufficient awareness levels especially among women vis-à-vis HIV/AIDS, even in a highly literate state such as Goa, in present time of widespread 'exposure' and numerous awareness promoting state/NGO initiatives, studies such as Falleiro (2009) have shown inadequate awareness levels even when it comes to *educated* undergraduate college students in Goa. Incidentally, related to poor awareness levels among women, it has been found that the return on investment in women's education is higher than the return on educating men, with studies in Malaysia showing the net return to education at all levels of wages and productivity being

20 per cent higher for girls and young women than for their male counterparts; because of which the World Bank even offers in some countries financial assistance to parents who allow girl children to go to school (Reid 2000c: 783–784).

Education vaccine is probably the best protective barrier for HIV/AIDS prevention (Pradhan et al. 2006: 99). Education, inclusive of information, (education) and communication or IEC,[9] which is a key to an effective response to HIV/AIDS, could be provided via various ways, including having compulsory year-long modules for students on 'Sex Education' or 'Adolescence Life Skills' in formal educational settings (Falleiro 2010; WHO 1995: 36). The successful initiative in Tamil Nadu which worked through education and communication paradigms that bring changes in health care-seeking behaviour, besides engaging high-risk group members as community health personnel, could also assist in HIV prevention (Krishnamoorthy 2010: 9). Additionally, despite improvements in numbers of those testing for HIV, there is a need to create greater awareness since a large number of people are still unaware of their infected status. If fear and/or denial hold back people from knowing their status at an early stage of infection, the same needs to be overcome by effectively communicating the benefits that include delayed onset of AIDS and fewer chances of infecting others.[10] Additionally, knowledge of HIV status can help individuals/HHs to plan in advance for the future keeping in mind the progressively increasing need for more resources (Gupta 1998, in Gupta and Panda 2002: 192). Though preventive steps need to be focused on high-risk, vulnerable and low-income background sections, nevertheless those from the middle and upper middle class backgrounds too cannot be ignored just because they often remain invisible (Ramakrishna et al. 2008: 386). With HIV often becoming a lifestyle disease (Pereira 2008: 2), efforts towards prevention have to go beyond high-risk groups to even the massage and beauty parlours, discotheques, escort-providers, shacks, etc., dotting Goa's famous coastline, where incidentally HIV prevalence is among the highest.

Besides education, the other *preventive* way that can be adopted in the control of spread of HIV is providing safe blood/blood products, not just in Goa which is relatively better-off, but throughout the country on account of increasing inter-state movement of people. Blood transfusion has a very high HIV transmission rate of 90 per cent and above (Rao 2000c: 50; Sheth 2004: 27). With National Family Health Survey (NFHS–3) reporting 38–40 per cent of women in Goa being anaemic including pregnant/breastfeeding mothers, with the possibility that they may require blood transfusion, and since supply of blood by licensed commercial banks is only about 1/4th of the blood used in hospitals in India (see Medhini et al. 2007a: 46–47), attention still needs to be given to plug this mode of HIV transmission.

With regard to MTCT,[11] since there are about 30 per cent chances that the newborn will be HIV+ if the mother is (A. Kehra, in HRLN 2008: 30),[12] there is a need to plug this route of transmission[13] as well through adoption of educative programmes comprising of compulsory counselling sessions for expecting mothers and for couples before registration of marriage.[14] With perinatal transmission accounting for over 90 per cent of infections among infected children (Solomon et al. 2000: 99) and with HIV prevalence among women increasing to almost 50 per cent of all new infections, the sooner this route of transmission is taken care of, the better it will be to provide a brighter future for the children. Unfortunately in India, though ART for HIV+ pregnant women can reduce the risk of HIV transmission, over 75 per cent of the women are not on the same (Sinha 2008: 8; 2010b: 11).

5.2.2 'Curative' Measures

5.2.2A 'Medico-curative' Measures

Investment in health is a major asset not only in well-being but also in economic development; while poverty leads to bad health, bad health contributes to the continuation of poverty (Sachs 2008, 2). Treatment regimes and programmes need to be on a continuous and permanent basis especially considering that treatment is for the lifetime of PLWHA. Mere availability of health technologies is not enough; ensuring access to such technologies is critical (Gupta et al. 2007: 23). While proper treatment can improve the lives of those infected and affected themselves, it will additionally help at the sectoral and macro levels too.[15] The introduction of *highly active ART* (HAART) and availability of drugs for OIs has led to a decline in HIV/AIDS mortality. However, interrelated factors determine access to essential drugs, including cost, supply management, drug selection, legislation/regulation, manufacturing constraints, and R&D decisions (Medhini et al. 2007a: 139). Although the *first-line* ART is available and relatively inexpensive, for most Indians it is still costly and unaffordable, especially if one adds the cost of travel and need for frequent check-ups; in case of children it is far worse, with ART often costing up to 10 times as much as that for adults (ibid.: 109 and 570). Among others, the following measures could improve the 'treatment' aspect of HIV/AIDS:

- Taking care of the often-seen-in-India scenario of dilapidated state of infrastructure, poor quality/supply of drugs/ equipment and employee absenteeism especially at rural health centres (see also Panagariya 2008: 16) which has a negative effect on the sick, both, to go for treatment and to continue the same on a regular basis.
- While the *second-line* treatment should be provided/extended without delay,[16,17] since many on the *first-line* are resistant to the same especially due to poor adherence;[18] dispensing the *first-line* treatment itself should be streamlined with possibly more *link-ART centres* to cater to those living in the periphery. This could reduce grueling travelling ordeals for the PLWHA and improve adherence to treatment. Timely taken ART, besides improving the lifespan and well being, could keep PLWHA productive for more years, minimize impact on family earnings and help raise lifetime HH income (Bell et al. 2004: 124). Streamlining ART distribution could encourage needy PLWHA to avail of the same.
- Discrimination in health care settings (both public and private) should be done away with. The proposed legislation, the draft National Health Bill, 2009, which hinges on people's

participation and involvement in health issues, and which highlights patients rights and government obligations that no one is denied health in public/private hospitals, besides envisaging monitoring/redressal systems (Rajadhyaksha 2009: 1), should be vigorously pursued. To reduce medical discrimination, provisions need to be incorporated and invoked to suspend licenses of doctors/clinics involved in discrimination against PLWHA.

- Ensuring that the relatively new initiative of the government to provide free medication for OIs (Nair 2008b: 5) holds true for all illnesses/treatments, times and public health centres without exception; with patients especially from weaker sections not having to incur any personal expenses on treatment/medication.
- Averting delays and harrowing experiences at the ART centres; there should be alternative plans of action for any eventuality, including breakdown of CD-4 count equipment.
- Efforts should go to provide fair price health care and thus greater health equity, with mechanisms framed so that anyone could enter into any registered health care provider (private, NGO or state) and expect a proportional health care cost subsidy based on one's ability to pay (Krishnamoorthy 2009: 9). Private and NGO providers should enter to cover regions that lack public health care provision (ibid.).
- Concessional bus/railway passes should be made available to PLWHA, at least from poorer backgrounds, to travel for the purpose of seeking treatment. Besides reducing the hardships on HHs, this will as well help improve adherence to treatment.[19]
- Gender biases against females, whether in HHs or health care settings, should be done away with a multipronged strategy that includes incentives and explicit government support. Unfortunately, in the words of Delhi High Court Justice Muralidhar, 'Women (*often*) carry the burden of poverty in that they have to prove their "below poverty line" (BPL) status when trying to access health facilities' (Garg 2010: 8).

- An advisory should be handed to employers to provide relaxations in leave and/or hours of duty to HIV+ individuals to receive ART treatment and for employed HH members from HIV/AIDS HHs to perform caregiving duties.
- ARV drugs must be provided free to any accredited doctor even in the private sector. This will prevent chances of potential corruption in trying to sell drugs from the public sector to the private; and also prevent PLWHA from taking their drugs from public centres and going for guidance to the private sector. This can additionally assist to regulate doctors who gave incorrect care in the past (Pandey 2006: 13–14).
- PLWHA need to strictly adhere to their treatment regimen, with failure to do so having serious and possibly irreversible consequences: on the health, line of treatment and expense fronts. One of the ways that could be conveniently used to remind the HIV+ persons about their treatment/dosage is through the use of mobile phone short message service (SMS) or alerts, as has been done in a number of places in Africa, besides been arranged for in Goa as well by the state-run GSACS.[20]

In fine, notwithstanding that the right to health in all forms and levels should always contain elements of availability, accessibility, acceptability and quality (Medhini et al. 2007a: 7), for the greater, all-round and long-term good, we need to do away with the illusions of curative medicine, the *medicalization* of medical health, the use of urgency-driven curative medical solutions, the reduction of public health to bio-medical health, and mistaking primary care for public health (Jacob 2007: 10). Instead, among others, we need to focus on public health in terms of national interest, social justice and egalitarian society; with provision/access to water, sanitation, housing, nutrition, education and employment as basic rights (ibid.). Additionally, the principles guiding the 'treat 3 million by 2005' ('3 by 5') programme of WHO, namely: urgency, added value, integrated approach, partnership building and treatment as a human right (Narain and Gilks 2004: 112), could be used as standard guidelines by all for dispensing health services to PLWHA.

5.2.2B 'General Curative' Measures

- Gender inequality and poor respect for human rights of women, key factors in the HIV/AIDS epidemic from the viewpoint of effectiveness and social justice (Medhini et al. 2007a: 449), have to be wiped out immediately. Appropriate mechanisms have to be secured to prevent women from being exploited, victimized, thrown out from homes, besides having laws to safeguard their rights over property. Having laws *per se* may not suffice; they have to be publicized, with free legal services also provided (see also Dixit 2005: 90–92). 'Sensitiveness to individualization' could greatly help PLWHA in general and women in particular; the same could even help take care of suicidal tendencies (Thomas et al. 1997: 93–95), existence of which was revealed by the present study as well.

- Education, employment generation schemes, credit and social investment schemes, etc., to be looked as redistributive mechanisms to address critical needs and improve human conditions (Reid 2000c: 783). In recent times, some NGOs have floated schemes for HIV/AIDS individuals/HHs towards capacity building by providing financial support to start home-based entrepreneurship programmes such as tailoring. Despite hardships faced at the time of availing the subsidy and post-subsidy, similar initiatives could be expanded to cover the entire state/country and all HIV/AIDS individuals/HHs after ironing out existing flaws. Initiatives towards the economic empowerment of HIV/AIDS infected/affected through measures such as providing assistance in getting bank loans to take up jobs and improve life as done by the Bellary District AIDS Prevention Society (BDAPS) in association with UNDP (Ahiraj 2007: 6) should be adopted by other regions as well to suit local needs. Encouraging and providing assistance towards capacity building and starting of self-help groups can help HIV/AIDS HHs in general and those headed by females in particular.

- To assist PLWHA to ease HH expenses and facilitate travel needs, the concessions promised by the Indian Railways should be provided not only for those on ART or those who seek treatment, but also to the economically vulnerable, to travel anywhere within the country for any purpose at least once a year. Likewise, state-owned bus services should provide concessional travel not only to the PLWHA, but also to children and HH members, at least of those who are in the advanced stages of infection and living below the poverty line.

- The economically poorer PLWHA based on economic conditions and/or stage of infection should be provided graded monthly pension/dole. While the model adopted by the government of Goa in providing the monthly sum to the HIV+ individuals through the Dayanand Social Security Scheme (DSSS) should be adopted by other states as well, in Goa itself, despite the welcome initiative, the amount provided should be periodically raised in view of rise in the cost of living. Hurdles faced by PLWHA vis-à-vis documentation procedures (such as getting income/residence certificates) need to be appropriate addressed with a humane face. As initiated in Odisha,[21] besides pension to PLWHA, monetary assistance has to be provided to AIDS widows as well (Mohanty 2008: 12).

- Food assistance and security has to be assured by the government. The initiative started by Goa Agriculture Department through the Goa State Horticulture Corporation Limited (GSHCL) to provide subsidized commodities through mobile vans and vegetable outlets should increasingly cover slum areas and places where there are known pockets of PLWHA. The promise by the Centre to HIV+ individuals to provide job cards/employment under the National Rural Employment Guarantee Act (NREGA), besides being treated as belonging to BPL category and ensuring them 35 kg of food grain every month under the *Antyodaya Anna Yojana* (AAY) scheme (Mahapatra 2008: 1 and 7) should be fulfilled without any exceptions, delays and bureaucratic/political hurdles. The 'Right to Food' as assured by the United Progressive Alliance-II (UPA-II) government at the Centre, though not particularly aimed at PLWHA, could be of much assistance since it envisages subsidized community kitchens for homeless and migrants; guaranteed access to sufficient food especially for vulnerable sections; and 25 kg of rice or wheat per month at ₹3 per kg to BPL families.

- Schemes such as those started by the Directorate of Women and Child Development under the *Vatra Bhet* scheme wherein a *saree* and dress material is distributed as New Year gift to BPL women housed in registered shelters and children in *Apna Ghar* (Goa), should be extended to all HIV+ women and children from BPL HHs.

- Insurance companies should be encouraged to provide *cover* to PLWHA since many, especially from the better economic backgrounds, though desirous for insurance cover, are denied of the same because of being infected. To PLWHA from lower economic backgrounds, insurance cover should be provided as done by the pilot initiative of group insurance plan introduced in Karnataka by Population Services International (PSI) in partnership with Star Health and Allied Insurance Company and the Karnataka Network for Positive People (KNP+), which besides covering treatment costs, provides ₹30,000 insurance cover; with ₹15,000 being provided for hospitalization and an equal amount provided to the family in case of death.

- Discrimination at the workplace should be made a serious and punishable offence. Termination of a PLWHA (who are appropriately qualified and functionally capable of doing the job and who pose no risk to others vis-à-vis transmission of HIV) should be strictly prohibited. The same criteria need to be applied at the time of applying for and filling of new jobs as well. Those currently employed who fail the above-mentioned pre-conditions should be provided suitable alternative employment instead of being made to leave the job. Alternative job as compassionate employment should be provided as a right or priority to HH members of those PLWHA who need to be terminated or released from employment due to incapability of work. Providing a job to a family member of an HIV+ person as rehabilitation should not be at the cost of exploitation of the person (Chopra 2008: 13).

- Free legal services provided by NGOs, such as HRLN and Lawyers Collective, to defend and protect PLWHA against discrimination or denial by defending their basic right to life and health; to take litigation of HIV-infected/affected persons for court/out-of-court settlements; to take matters of public concern to higher authorities; to increase awareness of legal rights and remedies, etc., should be extended and widely publicized so that benefits reach even the illiterate and less educated, and those in the unorganized and informal sectors.
- Since HIV/AIDS epidemic cannot be tackled by the government alone, it is critical for other sectors, including individuals, HHs, NGOs and the corporate sector to also contribute. Pooling resources, financial and otherwise, is going to be necessary, especially if long-term sustainability of intervention efforts is to be met.

In fine, to improve the economic well-being of PLWHA, we need to effectively follow the Chinese programme of 'Four Frees and One Care': *free* ART, voluntary counselling/testing, drugs to prevent MTCT and schooling for (orphaned) children; and economic assistance to affected HHs. While in Goa and parts of India, we may be doing relatively well vis-à-vis the 'four frees', we need to do much more on the complex issue of 'one care'. To improve the economic well-being of PLWHA and their families, we need to see that the inglorious history of NACP-II, as per the *Detailed Implementation Review* of the World Bank[22] (in Jain 2008b: 1–2) and NACO[23] (in Chatterjee and Sahgal 2002: 63–64) does not repeat itself.

Notes

1. Diabetes, for example, was to 'bleed India of US$32 billion...' during the year (Sinha 2010a: 9).
2. Though the poor should not be denied access to essential medicines, even in the USA, as reported earlier by Kakar and Kakar (2001: 269), the benefit of HAART had not reached all segments of the population.
3. Among the market failures, while the first involves under-provision of public good, specifically the lack of incentives for the private sector to collect and/

or disseminate information; the second involves negative externalities of high-risk behaviour; and the third involves equity, with very poor people being less able to protect themselves against HIV than others (Israni 2001). According to Drummond and Kelly (2006: 11–13), while one failure is the continued lack of education, with many ignorant of AIDS being incapable of protecting themselves from HIV; a second is that adequate health care supplies for prevention/treatment do not reach those most likely to benefit; with those who are at risk generally being the least able to afford medications.

4. Preventive measures have been provided for their 'indirect' role in tackling the adverse economic fallouts—that is, by averting contraction of HIV infection itself.

5. So that accompanying adverse economic fallouts are taken care of.

6. To substantiate, take examples of employment and education: while having an appropriate job *ante*-HIV could provide support to HHs, thereby *preventing* individuals from going to 'HIV-risky' avenues such as prostitution; providing assured employment to HIV+ individuals/other HH members post HIV is important to sustain HHs. Likewise, while education *ante*-HIV can make people aware of the modes of HIV transmission/prevention besides making people more capable for employment; education post HIV, despite HIV imposed pressures to discontinue, ensures an optimistic future for children.

7. Centre where free counseling and testing for HIV is done and basic information on modes of HIV transmission and prevention provided. Additionally, these centres link people to other prevention, care and treatment services; provide drugs for OIs; and follow-up counselling through field visits. There were as of December 2009, 14 ICTCs with three private hospitals also added to the list (Nagarsekar 2009: 7).

8. See Chapter 11: http://www.nfhsindia.org/chapters.html, accessed January 2009.

9. IEC is a process that informs, motivates and helps people to adopt and maintain healthy practices and life skills. It aims at empowering individuals and enabling them to make correct decisions about safe behaviours/practices (*TOI* 1 December 2008; see also Rao 2000b: 547).

10. See 'A pioneering effort on HIV', *The Hindu*, Karnataka, 20 November 2007, 8.

11. This vertical form of HIV transmission includes *ante*-, *intra*- and post-partum transmission.

12. 10 to 50 per cent according to Pande (2000: 117).

13. Standard medical alternatives are available to minimize the risks to bare minimum levels.

14. Incidentally, in the context of registration of marriage, with the urgent need to contain the spread of HIV/AIDS and its serious fallouts, as mentioned in *Chapter 1* various state governments in India including Goa had shown intent to make HIV testing compulsory for couples before registration of marriage. Though the same has not yet become a firm policy measure in Goa (on account of various contentious issues); efforts are nevertheless being made by some such as the Catholic Church to educate couples (before marriage) on HIV/AIDS during the compulsory *Marriage Formation Course*. Such initiatives, if followed by others as well, could contribute positively in arresting the spread of HIV.

15. A study in South Africa indicated that if half of those needing ART are provided the same, the effect of HIV on economic growth would be reduced by 17 per cent (Fredricksson and Kanabus 2007).
16. At around the time of this study, those PLWHA from Goa who were to be on it, were referred to Mumbai, Maharashtra, some 350 km away from Goa, that too one way!
17. Currently NACO is focusing more on the *first-line* treatment by even refusing the *second-line* ART to those who received the *first-line* in private hospitals by citing the following: low prevalence of HIV in India; less allocation of grants from Global Fund for Care, Support and Treatment (GFCST); greater focus on prevention programmes instead of care and treatment; cost of one *second-line* treatment being equal to the *first-line* treatment of six patients and TB treatment of 25 (Mahapatra 2010: 8).
18. See 'Now, HIV therapy in 8 more states', *TOI*, Goa, 5 January 2009, 7.
19. Indian Railways should honour their announced plan without delay to provide 75 per cent concession to PLWHA, in line with that existing for cancer patients, for seeking treatment (Rao 2008: 9).
20. See http://www.firstpost.com/fwire/now-goa-govt-to-remind-hiv-patients-of-their-dosage-through-sms-470309.html. Also see http://www.akvo.org/rsr/project/554/ (both accessed on March 2013).
21. Though initiative was good, it needs to be nevertheless relooked into, to see whether amount provided is sufficient considering the prevailing cost of living.
22. Involving salaries of fictitious people, unqualified NGOs pulling strings, government officers getting cuts to award contracts and politicians acting as middlemen in bribery.
23. *Alleged* to have become the casualty of political interference, with guidelines often ignored and resulting in setbacks to NGO participation. While in several states less than 10 per cent of the funds were utilized in certain years; excluding exceptions, empowered committees were either not constituted or were left sidelined; with low level NGO participation ruling out sustained experimentation with innovative approaches.

Appendix I

Sample Profile

Table AI.i

Profile of HIV/AIDS sample HHs

	Frequency	Per cent		Frequency	Per cent
Place of origin of the HIV/AIDS HH head			**Location of HIV/AIDS HHs**		
Goa	90	45	Urban	94	47
Outside Goa	110	55	Rural	106	53
Total	**200**	**100**	**Total**	**200**	**100**
District-wise HIV/AIDS HHs distribution			**Sex of HIV/AIDS HH head**		
North Goa	92	46	Male	117	58.5
South Goa	108	54	Female	83	41.5
Total	**200**	**100**	**Total**	**200**	**100**
Taluka-wise HIV/AIDS HHs distribution			**Religion of the HIV/AIDS HH head**		
Bardez	37	18.5	Catholic	50	25
Tiswadi	18	9	Hindu	124	62
Ponda	22	11	Muslim	21	10.5
Marmagoa	52	26	Others	5	2.5
Salcete	45	22.5	**Total**	**200**	**100**
Others (six talukas)	26	13	**Place of obtaining information**		
Total	**200**	**100**	Respondents homes: 15%; C&S Homes: 21.5%;Drop-in-Centre's/ NGO premises: 58%; Others: 5.5%		

Source: Author's field work.

Table AI.ii

Comparative profile of sample HHs based on profile of HH head and total annual HH income

(*figures in percentage terms given in brackets*)

	HIV/AIDS HHs			Non-HIV/AIDS HHs		
	Sex of HH head			Sex of HH head		
	Male	Female	Total	Male	Female	Total
Age of the HH head						
20–30 years	6 (3)	13 (6.5)	19 (9.5)	6 (3)	2 (1)	8 (4)
31–40 years	49 (24.5)	28 (14)	77 (38.5)	34 (17)	14 (7)	48 (24)
41–50 years	32 (16)	15 (7.5)	47 (23.5)	53 (26.5)	15 (7.5)	68 (34)
51–60 years	20 (10)	17 (8.5)	37 (18.5)	42 (21)	10 (5)	52 (26)
Above 60 years	10 (5)	10 (5)	20 (10)	17 (8.5)	7 (3.5)	24 (12)
Educational qualifications of the HH head						
Illiterate	27 (13.5)	47 (23.5)	74 (37)	37 (18.5)	33 (16.5)	70 (35)
Primary	13 (6.5)	10 (5)	23 (11.5)	32 (16)	5 (2.5)	37 (18.5)
Fifth to SSC	57 (28.5)	20 (10)	77 (38.5)	69 (34.5)	10 (5)	79 (39.5)
HSSC	8 (4)	2 (1)	10 (5)	10 (5)	0	10 (5)
Graduate	9 (4.5)	3 (1.5)	12 (6)	3 (1.5)	0	3 (1.5)
Postgraduate	1 (.5)	0	1 (.5)	0	0	0
Others	2 (1)	1 (.5)	3 (1.5)	1 (.5)	0	1 (.5)

(Table AI.ii Continued)

(Table AI.ii Continued)

| | HIV/AIDS HHs | | | Non-HIV/AIDS HHs | | |
| | Sex of HH head | | | Sex of HH head | | |
	Male	Female	Total	Male	Female	Total
Earning category of the HH head						
Salary earner	36 (18)	10 (5)	46 (23)	50 (25)	4 (2)	54 (27)
Wage earner	26 (13)	23 (11.5)	49 (24.5)	65 (32.5)	22 (11)	87 (43.5)
Self employed	16 (8)	5 (2.5)	21 (10.5)	13 (6.5)	2 (1)	15 (7.5)
Not applicable*	39 (19.5)	45 (22.5)	84 (42)	24 (12)	20 (10)	44 (22)
Total annual HH-income						
Up to ₹25,000	25 (12.5)	32 (16)	57 (28.5)	1 (.5)	2 (1)	3 (1.5)
₹25,001–50,000	35 (17.5)	36 (18)	71 (35.5)	18 (9)	20 (10)	38 (19)
₹50,001–1,00,000	33 (16.5)	9 (4.5)	42 (21)	60 (30)	12 (6)	72 (36)
₹1,00,001–1,50,000	11 (5.5)	3 (1.5)	14 (7)	35 (17.5)	8 (4)	43 (21.5)
₹1,50,001–2,00,000	6 (3)	1 (.5)	7 (3.5)	26 (13)	2 (1)	28 (14)
₹2,00,001–2,50,000	1 (.5)	1 (.5)	2 (1)	5 (2.5)	2 (1)	7 (3.5)
₹2,50,001–3,00,000	0	0	0	2 (1)	0	2 (1)
₹3,00,001–5,00,000	5 (2.5)	1 (.5)	6 (3)	5 (2.5)	2 (1)	7 (3.5)
Above ₹5,00,000	1 (.5)	0	1 (.5)	0	0	0
Total	117 (58.5)	83 (41.5)	200 (100)	152 (76)	48 (24)	200 (100)

Source: Author's field work.

Note: *Non-earning members on account of unemployment, sickness, being housewives, retired, etc.

Table AI.iii

Comparative profile of sample HHs on the basis of employment of HH heads

(figures in percentage terms given in brackets)

Occupation of the HH head	HIV/AIDS HHs			Non-HIV/AIDS HHs		
	Sex of HH head			Sex of HH head		
	Male	*Female*	*Total*	*Male*	*Female*	*Total*
Farmer/cultivator	1 (.5)	0	1 (.5)	2 (1)	0	2 (1)
Agricultural labour	1 (.5)	0	1 (.5)	10 (5)	1 (.5)	11 (5.5)
Construction/related work	10 (5)	3 (1.5)	13 (6.5)	31 (15.5)	8 (4)	39 (19.5)
Skilled/semi-skilled/non-agricultural labour	22 (11)	3 (1.5)	25 (12.5)	35 (17.5)	1 (.5)	36 (18)
Service (government/private)	21 (10.5)	9 (4.5)	30 (15)	29 (14.5)	6 (3)	35 (17.5)
Petty business/small shop	7 (3.5)	5 (2.5)	12 (6)	7 (3.5)	1 (.5)	8 (4)
Small artisan in household/cottage industry	0	1 (.5)	1 (.5)	0	0	0
Self employed/professional	3 (1.5)	0	3 (1.5)	1 (.5)	2 (1)	3 (1.5)
Truck driver/cleaner	5 (2.5)	0	5 (2.5)	4 (2)	0	4 (2)
Other kind of driver	4 (2)	0	4 (2)	8 (4)	0	8 (4)
Pensioner/retired	14 (7)	11 (5.5)	25 (12.5)	21 (10.5)	3 (1.5)	24 (12)
Domestic servant/housemaids	3 (1.5)	17 (8.5)	20 (10)	0	9 (4.5)	9 (4.5)
Rentier/house	0	1 (.5)	1 (.5)	0	0	0
Housewife	0	17 (8.5)	17 (8.5)	0	17 (8.5)	17 (8.5)

(Table AI.iii Continued)

(Table A1.iii Continued)

	HIV/AIDS HHs			Non-HIV/AIDS HHs		
	Sex of HH head			Sex of HH head		
	Male	Female	Total	Male	Female	Total
Unemployed	1 (.5)	0	1 (.5)	2 (1)	0	2 (1)
Sick—cannot work	25 (12.5)	16 (8)	41 (20.5)	2 (1)	0	2 (1)
Total	**117 (58.5)**	**83 (41.5)**	**200 (100)**	**152 (76)**	**48 (24)**	**200 (100)**
Sector of employment of the HH head (*if employed only*)						
Agriculture/allied activities	2 (1)	0	2 (1)	13 (6.5)	0	13 (6.5)
Mining/quarrying	0	1 (.5)	1 (.5)	1 (.5)	0	1 (.5)
Manufacturing	1 (.5)	1 (.5)	2 (1)	3 (1.5)	1 (.5)	4 (2)
Construction	19 (9.5)	3 (1.5)	22 (11)	54 (27)	9 (4.5)	63 (31.5)
Trade	13 (6.5)	7 (3.5)	20 (10)	11 (5.5)	4 (2)	15 (7.5)
Transport/storage/communication	10	0	10 (5)	12 (6)	0	12 (6)
Hotel/restaurant	12 (6)	1 (.5)	13 (6.5)	5 (2.5)	1 (.5)	6 (3)
Finance/insurance/real estate/business services	3 (1.5)	0	3 (1.5)	1 (.5)	0	1 (.5)
Health	0	1 (.5)	1 (.5)	1 (.5)	0	1 (.5)
Community/social/personal services	16 (8)	24 (12)	40 (20)	16 (8)	13 (6.5)	29 (14.5)
Others (including government administration)	1 (.5)	0	1 (.5)	10 (5)	0	10 (5)
Total *	**77 (38.5)**	**38 (19)**	**115 (57.5)**	**127 (63.5)**	**28 (14)**	**155 (77.5)**

Source: Author's field work.

Note: The remaining 42.5 per cent and 22.5 per cent from the total HIV/AIDS and non-HIV/AIDS HHs respectively are currently not working due to unemployment, sickness, being housewives, retired, etc.

Table AI.iv

Employment and educational qualifications of HH members excluding the HH head

	HIV/AIDS HHs		Non-HIV/AIDS HHs	
	Frequency	*Per cent*	*Frequency*	*Per cent*
'Highest category' occupation of any HH member excluding the HH head in terms of earnings/designation/nature of job				
Farmer/cultivator	0	0	2	1
Agricultural labourer	1	.5	2	1
Construction	4	2	6	3
Skilled/semi-skilled/non-agricultural labourer	15	7.5	11	5.5
Service (government/private)	24	12	33	16.5
Petty business/small shop	3	1.5	4	2
Large business/medium-large shop	1	.5	0	0
Self employed/professional	1	.5	0	0
Truck driver/cleaner	3	1.5	1	.5
Transport worker	5	2.5	2	1
Domestic servant	12	6.0	9	4.5
Sub-total	*69*	*34.5*	*70*	*35*
HHs where no one has 'better' job than HH head	131	65.5	130	65
Sector of employment of the above member				
Agriculture/allied	1	.5	4	2
Manufacturing	4	2	5	2.5
Construction	8	4	12	6
Trade	7	3.5	8	4
Transport/storage/communication	9	4.5	5	2.5
Hotel/restaurant	6	3	2	1
Finance/insurance/real estate/ business services	2	1	1	.5
Community/social/personal services	27	13.5	29	14.5
Tourism	1	.5	0	0
Others (including government)	4	2	4	2
Sub-total	*69*	*34.5*	*70*	*35*
Not applicable	131	65.5	130	65

(Table AI.iv Continued)

(Table AI.iv Continued)

	HIV/AIDS HHs		Non-HIV/AIDS HHs	
	Frequency	Per cent	Frequency	Per cent
Highest educational qualifications attained in the HH excluding that of the HH head				
Primary	6	3	7	3.5
Fifth to SSC	55	27.5	47	23.5
HSSC	15	7.5	43	21.5
Graduate	9	4.5	28	14
Postgraduate	3	1.5	4	2
Professional	0	0	1	.5
Diploma	4	2	3	1.5
Sub-total	*92*	*46*	*133*	*66.5*
HHs where no one has better educational qualifications than HH head	108	54	67	33.5
Total	**200**	**100**	**200**	**100**

Source: Author's field work.

Table AI.v

Descriptive statistics of sample HHs

	HIV/AIDS HHs					Non-HIV/AIDS HHs				
	Min	Max	Sum of all HHs	Mean	SD	Min	Max	Sum of all HHs	Mean	SD
Age of HH head (years)	22	85	–	44.95	12.82	25	83	–	48.42	10.71
Size of the HH	1	11	754*	3.77	1.86	1	9	895	4.48	1.50
No. of non-working members in HH	.00	8	521	2.61	1.65	.00	7	534	2.67	1.40
Total no. of literate members in HH	.00	8	490	2.45	1.41	.00	7	587	2.94	1.50

Source: Author's field work.
Note: *Of this figure, 304 members were having confirmed HIV+ status.

Table AI.vi

Comparative profile of sample HHs on the basis of basic facilities used

(percentage figures shown in brackets)

	HIV/AIDS HHs			Non-HIV/AIDS HHs		
	Sex of HH head			*Sex of HH head*		
	Male	*Female*	*Total*	*Male*	*Female*	*Total*
Type of house						
Pucca	56 (28)	40 (20)	**96 (48)**	74 (37)	13 (6.5)	**87 (43.5)**
Semi-pucca	44 (22)	30 (15)	**74 (37)**	66 (33)	27 (13.5)	**93 (46.5)**
Kutcha	17 (8.5)	13 (6.5)	**30 (15)**	12 (6)	8 (4)	**20 (10)**
Electricity in the house						
Yes	110 (55)	75 (37.5)	**185 (92.5)**	144 (72)	48 (24)	**192 (96)**
No	7 (3.5)	8 (4)	**15 (7.5)**	8 (4)	0	**8 (4)**
Main source of drinking water						
Private tap	74 (37)	51 (25.5)	**125 (62.5)**	91 (45.5)	31 (15.5)	**122 (61)**
Public tap	20 (10)	13 (6.5)	**33 (16.5)**	26 (13)	9 (4.5)	**35 (17.5)**
Public hand pump	1 (.5)	1 (.5)	**2 (1)**	1 (.5)	0	**1 (.5)**
Tube well/private hand pump	5 (2.5)	2 (1)	**7 (3.5)**	4 (2)	1 (.5)	**5 (2.5)**
Own well	2 (1)	2 (1)	**4 (2)**	13 (6.5)	4 (2)	**17 (8.5)**
Public well	4 (2)	9 (4.5)	**13 (6.5)**	10 (5)	1 (.5)	**11 (5.5)**
River/pond	1 (.5)	0	**1 (.5)**	0	0	**0**
Others	10 (5)	5 (2.5)	**15 (7.5)**	7 (3.5)	2 (1)	**9 (4.5)**
Fuel used for cooking						
Firewood	19 (9.5)	18 (9)	**37 (18.5)**	38 (19)	17 (8.5)	**55 (27.5)**
Kerosene	28 (14)	15 (7.5)	**43 (21.5)**	20 (10)	8 (4)	**28 (14)**
LPG	67 (33.5)	50 (25)	**117 (58.5)**	94 (47)	23 (11.5)	**117 (58.5)**
Others	1 (.5)	0	**1 (.5)**	0	0	**0**
N.A. (No cooking)	2 (1)	0	**2 (1)**	0	0	**0**
Type of HH toilet						
No toilet*	27 (13.5)	35 (17.5)	**62 (31)**	41 (20.5)	25 (12.5)	**66 (33)**
Common toilet	33 (16.5)	10 (5)	**43 (21.5)**	25 (12.5)	7 (3.5)	**32 (16)**

(Table AI.vi Continued)

(Table AI.vi Continued)

	HIV/AIDS HHs			Non-HIV/AIDS HHs		
	Sex of HH head			Sex of HH head		
	Male	Female	Total	Male	Female	Total
Own toilet (flush)	47 (23.5)	31 (15.5)	**78 (39)**	64 (32)	12 (6)	**76 (38)**
Own toilet (traditional/pigs)	5 (2.5)	3 (1.5)	**8 (4)**	14 (7)	3 (1.5)	**17 (8.5)**
Sulabh toilet	5 (2.5)	4 (2)	**9 (4.5)**	8 (4)	1 (.5)	**9 (4.5)**
Total	**117 (58.5)**	**83 (41.5)**	**200 (100)**	**152 (76)**	**48 (24)**	**200 (100)**

Source: Author's field work.
Note: *These HHs make use of open/public areas for their needs.

Table AI.vii

Comparative profile of sample HHs based on ownership of items

(percentage figures shown in brackets)

	HIV/AIDS HHs		Non-HIV/AIDS HHs	
	Yes (HH owns)	No (HH does not own)	Yes (HH owns)	No (HH does not own)
Livestock	11 (5.5)	189 (94.5)	27 (13.5)	173 (86.5)
Radio/tape recorder/audio-set	88 (44)	112 (56)	128 (64)	72 (36)
Television	124 (62)	76 (38)	145 (72.5)	55 (27.5)
Refrigerator	63 (31.5)	137 (68.5)	79 (39.5)	121 (60.5)
Phone (landline)	29 (14.5)	171 (85.5)	52 (26)	148 (74)
Cell phone	144 (72)	56 (28)	148 (74)	52 (26)
Washing machine	15 (7.5)	185 (92.5)	31 (15.5)	169 (84.5)
Fan	162 (81)	38 (19)	178 (89)	22 (11)
Motorcycle	62 (31)	138 (69)	86 (43)	114 (57)
Own house/flat	102 (51)	98 (49)	143 (71.5)	57 (28.5)
Plot/land	37 (18.5)	163 (81.5)	54 (27)	146 (73)
Car/four-wheeler	8 (4)	192 (96)	13 (6.5)	187 (93.5)
Own well	10 (5)	190 (95)	27 (13.5)	173 (86.5)
AC	6 (3)	194 (97)	3 (1.5)	197 (98.5)
Computer	17 (8.5)	183 (91.5)	48 (24)	152 (76)

Source: Author's field work.

Table AI.viii

HIV status of HH head

(figures in brackets are percentage figures in terms of each category)

	Male HH head	Female HH head	Total
HH head **is** HIV+	87 (74.36)	52 (62.65)	**139 (69.5)**
HH head **does not have** HIV	30 (25.64)	31 (37.35)	**61 (30.5)**
Total	**117 (58.5)**	**83 (41.5)**	**200 (100)**

Source: Author's field work.

Table AI.ix

Profile of HIV+ respondents

(figures in brackets are percentage figures in terms of total sample)

	Male	Female	Total
Age-group of HIV+ respondents			
Below 30 years	12 (6)	46 (23)	**58 (29)**
31–40 years	41 (20.5)	46 (23)	**87 (43.5)**
41–50 years	26 (13)	16 (8)	**42 (21)**
51–60 years	11 (5.5)	2 (1)	**13 (6.5)**
HIV+ respondents: literate or illiterate			
Literate	78 (39)	77 (38.5)	**155 (77.5)**
Illiterate	12 (6)	33 (16.5)	**45 (22.5)**
Total	**90 (45)**	**110 (55)**	**200 (100)**
Marital status of HIV+ respondents			
Currently married	53 (26.5)	37 (18.5)	**90 (45)**
Separated/divorced/abandoned	8 (4)	11 (5.5)	**19 (9.5)**
Widowed	8 (4)	59 (29.5)	**67 (33.5)**
Unmarried	21 (10.5)	3 (1.5)	**24 (12)**
Nature of present earnings of HIV+ respondents			
Salary earner	37 (18.5)	19 (9.5)	**56 (28)**
Wage earner	14 (7)	27 (13.5)	**41 (20.5)**
Self employed	12 (6)	7 (3.5)	**19 (9.5)**

(Table AI.ix Continued)

(Table AI.ix Continued)

	Male	Female	Total
N.A. (currently unemployed/housewife/ retired/sick, etc.)	27 (13.5)	57 (28.5)	84 (42)
How HIV+ status was first discovered			
Voluntary testing*	36 (18)	55 (27.5)	91 (45.5)
After prolonged illness**	43 (21.5)	35 (17.5)	78 (39)
'Blood test'	10 (5)	5 (2.5)	15 (7.5)
During pregnancy	0	13 (6.5)	13 (6.5)
Others	1 (.5)	2 (1)	3 (1.5)
Number of years back HIV+ status detected			
1 year or less	21 (10.5)	22 (11)	43 (21.5)
1 year to 5 years	52 (26)	66 (33)	118 (59)
Over 5 years	17 (8.5)	22 (11)	39 (19.5)
Total	**90 (45)**	**110 (55)**	**200 (100)**

Source: Author's field work.

Notes: *With regard to voluntary testing, amongst others, the same was done by 47 respondents since spouse/partner was infected, with 32 doing on account of sickness-cum-suggestion of health provider, and/or since another HH member (not spouse) was infected.

**The prolonged illness was mostly fever (continuing for a long period of time), TB, skin infection/boils and vomiting/diarrhoea.

Table AI.x

Age description of sample HIV+ respondents

	Min.	Max.	Mean	SD
Age of the HIV+ respondents (years)	20	60	36.50	8.73

Source: Author's field work.

Appendix II

Income and Employment

Table AII.i

Age and employment of the dead AIDS members

	Frequency	Per cent figures for entire sample	Per cent figures for only those dead
Age-wise distribution of the dead AIDS members			
Below 18 years	5	2.5	6.5
18–30 years	22	11	28.6
31–40 years	35	17.5	45.5
41–50 years	12	6	15.6
51–60 years	3	1.5	3.9
Total—HHs of dead members	77	38.5	100
Others—that is, those who did not die	123	61.5	
Occupation of the dead AIDS members			
Farmer/cultivator	1	.5	1.3
Agricultural labourer	1	.5	1.3
Construction	17	8.5	22.1
Skilled/semi-skilled/non-agricultural labourer	20	10	26
Service (government/private)	8	4	10.4
Petty business/small shop	6	3	7.8
Self employed/professional	1	.5	1.3
Truck driver	4	2	5.2

(Table AII.i Continued)

(Table AII.i Continued)

	Frequency	Per cent figures for entire sample	Per cent figures for only those dead
Other transport worker	7	3.5	9.1
Domestic servant	2	1	2.6
Housewife	1	.5	1.3
Not working#	6	3	7.8
Others	3	1.5	3.9
Total—HHs of dead members	*77*	*38.5*	*100*
Others—that is, those who did not die	123	61.5	
Sector of employment of the above			
Agriculture/allied activities	2	1	2.6
Mining/quarrying	1	.5	1.3
Manufacturing	4	2	5.2
Construction	22	11	28.6
Trade	12	6	15.6
Transport/storage/ communication	12	6	15.6
Hotels/restaurants	7	3.5	9.1
Finance/insurance/real estate/ bus. services	1	.5	1.3
Health	1	.5	1.3
Community/social/personal services	1	.5	1.3
Others (including government service)	7	3.5	9.1
Non-working members	7	3.5	9.1
Total—HHs of dead members	*77*	*38.5*	*100*
Others—that is, those who did not die	123	61.5	
Total of all HHs	**200**	**100**	

Source: Author's field work.
Note: #Includes five minors.

Table AII.ii

*Summarized details of present and past employment status of CGs**

	Present status of CGs	*Past status of CGs*
Total no. of CGs employed at present: 38 [19%] (61.29%)	• No. of CGs who lost income last year: 30 [15%] *(78.95%)*	–
	• No. of CGs who did not lose income last year: 8 [4%] *(21.05%)*	–
Total no. of CGs unemployed at present: 24 [12%] (38.71%)	○ No. of CGs presently unemployed but were employed earlier: 6 [3%] *(25%)*	• Lost income: 4 [2%] *(66.67%)* • Did not lose income: 2 [1%] *(33.33)*
	○ No. of CGs unemployed at present and unemployed earlier: 15 [7.5%] *(62.5%)*	–
	○ N.A. (minors): 3 [1.5%] *(12.5%)*	–
Total: 62 [31%] (100%)	62 [31%] *(100%)*	6 [3%] *(100%)*

Source: Author's field work.
Note: *Percentage figures in square brackets "[ ]" represent total number of HHs, with italicized figures in round brackets "( )" representing percentage figures for the said category only.

Table AII.iii

Coping mechanisms adopted and total annual HH income slabs

Total annual HH income slabs	*Wife/HIV+ female respondent took up job*	*Minor children took up job*	*Those above 60 years took up job*	*HIV+ respondent took additional job*
Up to ₹25,000	11	5	1	1
₹25,001–50,000	22	6	4	8
₹50,001–1,00,000	6	1	4	2
₹1,00,001–1,50,000	2	1	1	1
₹1,50,001–2,00,000	1	0	0	0
₹2,00,001–2,50,000	0	0	0	0
₹2,50,001–3,00,000	0	0	0	0
₹3,00,001–5,00,000	2	0	0	0
Above ₹5,00,000	0	0	0	0
Total	**44**	**13**	**10**	**12**

Source: Author's field work.

Appendix III

About the Study

Study Objectives

To get the challenging and overwhelming economic impact of HIV/AIDS on individuals/HHs addressed effectively, it is necessary to first understand and document the factual day-to-day living conditions and ground realities facing the infected and affected; without a comprehensive study, neither will the quantum nor the nature of relief measures needed be known. The primary objective of the present study was the systematic documentation of the economic impact of HIV/AIDS on individuals/HHs. The areas extensively researched were: the impact of HIV/AIDS on income and employment; the impact of HIV/AIDS on the inflow and outflow of HH income; and the impact of HIV/AIDS on health and medical expenditures. To understand the intricacies of these impacts, two sets of comparative analyses were made: a gender-based analysis and an analysis involving a matched sample of non-HIV/AIDS HHs. Unless specified, the focus of the present study (vis-à-vis objectives) in the context of the time period was the 'last one year' (that is, 12 months preceding the present study) or the 'last one month' (that is, 30 days preceding the study).

Research Design, Methodology and Sample Profile

1. **Population:** The true *universe* of HIV+ individuals is unknown because of reasons ranging from infected individuals not having tested themselves, to individuals, especially from better income brackets, who test themselves in private clinics or outside the state and do not reveal their HIV+ status. Considering the above, for the purpose of the present study, the sample was drawn from a *working* universe covering both districts of Goa and comprising HIV+ persons within the age group of 18–60 years, whose HIV+ status was detected/registered in Goa at the ICTCs as on 31 December 2008 (as per official figures there were a total of about 11,674 HIV+ cases in Goa as on this date). Additionally, while only those who have a 'proper' place to stay (owned or rented) were considered for study; those living on railway platforms, in brothels, bus terminuses, public gardens, footpaths and such places 'outside' were excluded (since the study was on the impact of HIV/AIDS on individuals as members of HHs). Foreigners and residents of other states registered at the ICTCs in Goa have also been excluded.

    For the purpose of selecting the control group of non-HIV/AIDS HHs, the population comprised of HHs from both districts of Goa, having no member tested as HIV+, and which have a similar background as the HIV/AIDS HHs sample: background particularly with reference to educational qualifications and place of origin of the HH head, and locale and socio-cultural background of the HH. HHs having member(s) with critical life-debilitating medical ailments such as cancer were excluded for the purpose of defining the working population. The selection of non-HIV/AIDS HHs sample was based on inputs from PLWHA, NGOs, community leaders, social workers, among others. Only adult members having knowledge of the realities of the HHs were considered for the purpose of the interview. Interviews were done with the consent of respondents.

2. **Sampling procedure:** Although all HH members including HIV+ members were part of the study, the focus was on one HIV+ person per HH within the age group of 18–60 years. Considering that the universe of HIV+ individuals is unknown and that the study dealt with a highly sensitive issue involving hidden population, stigma, discrimination and non-disclosure of HIV+ status, a combination of non-probability sampling techniques were adopted including purposive, quota, snowball and convenience sampling techniques. Personal biases were avoided and elements of randomness used to minimize avoidable bias and unrepresentativeness of the sample.

Two major procedures were adopted to select the study sample. In the first, after highlighting the various aspects/objectives of the study, different NGOs/C&S Homes were requested to prepare a list of potential respondents from among their registered clients. The list was prepared keeping in mind the respondent's profile such as gender, economic background, religion, occupation, etc., and after verifying whether they were able and willing to be part of the study. From this list, where possible, sample respondents were chosen randomly. The sampling procedure was done largely through the assistance of NGOs since a free list/sampling frame of PLWHA is publicly unavailable. The second major method adopted for sample selection was that on any given day all those admitted or visiting C&S Homes and Drop-in-Centres were chosen, after explaining the study to them, obtaining their consent and clarifying about their right not to take part; if they qualified for the study, the exclusions and their disposition were also kept in mind.

The final sample whose details have been used for the purpose of analysis comprises of 200 HIV+ respondents representing 200 HHs. To corroborate the findings, to get additional inputs and to understand the finer nuances of the matter, especially since the study deals with a sensitive issue involving hidden population, a variation of the Focus Group Discussion (FGD) was used wherein discussions were held with groups of members comprising PLWHA as well as NGO counsellors and field workers. Similar to the sample of HIV/AIDS HHs, the control group also consisted of 200 HHs.

3. **Instrumentation:** The study made use of two separate questionnaires/schedules (Q-S): one for HIV/AIDS individuals/HHs and the other for the control group. These instruments were adapted from the ones prepared by NCAER (2004; Pradhan et al. 2006).

4. **Ethical considerations:** The study adheres to the basic principles of social research (see Neuman 2000: 102). Expected and accepted ethical norms were scrupulously followed.

5. **Data collection:** The interviews were done at/close to respondents' residence, at NGO premises, Drop-in-Centres or C&S Homes, with the support of doctors and NGO counsellors/field workers. Data collection was done between March and August 2009. To cross-check responses for authenticity, besides the Q-S itself being designed for the same, whenever possible the following steps were also taken: (i) other family members were questioned separately; (ii) verification of responses was done with members of NGOs/C&S Homes or doctors who were in contact with the respondents; and (3) verifying expense figures with bills/cash memos. To keep a check on the possibility of respondents inflating consumption expenditure and subduing income figures, matching of cash inflow with outflow was also done.

6. **Data methods and techniques:** Statistical tools such as mean and standard deviation (SD) and tests such as correlation, chi-square and Mann-Whitney U were used for data interpretation and analyses. While in case of correlation, Spearman's rank correlation and Kendall's tau rank correlation were adopted on account of the nature of the study; with regard to chi-square, Fisher's Exact Test was used whenever appropriate.

7. **About the sample:** Self-explanatory tables of the study samples are provided under Appendix I. While most HIV/AIDS HH-heads were from lower age groups, with the youngest being just 22 years old (mean age: 44.95 years) reflective of death, disbanding and/or dissolution of HHs on account of HIV/AIDS, it was the reverse for non-HIV/AIDS HHs, with most belonging to higher age brackets (mean age: 48.42 years). The average size of non-HIV/AIDS HHs was bigger at 4.48 members as opposed to 3.77 in case of the HIV/AIDS HHs. In case of 69.5 per cent HIV/AIDS HHs, HH-heads themselves were HIV+. The mean age of the HIV+ sample respondents was 36.5 years. While HIV/AIDS HHs were mostly from lower-income brackets, it was not the case with their matched counterparts who were relatively better-off. In consonance with other studies (see Dixit 2005: 111 and 142) there were more female-headed, often widow-led, HIV/AIDS HHs (83 as compared to 48 in non-HIV/AIDS HHs), with there being more male-headed non-HIV/AIDS HHs. The study revealed that being widowed mothers at the age of 21 is not uncommon in HIV/AIDS HHs; in one case a widow aged 20 years lived with four children.

Limitations

- The study deals with an extremely sensitive issue. Despite precautions taken, the accuracy of the profile prepared and the data analysis depend primarily on the information provided by the respondents.
- Considering the nature of the study, it is not possible to gain sufficient access to HIV+ individuals of all economic backgrounds, especially those from the better income brackets. Though in line with vast literature on the concentration of HIV/AIDS among poorer sections, and also despite broadly reflective of the types of HIV+ individuals listed at the ICTCs, there is the possibility that the sample may appear tilted towards those from lower economic backgrounds.

- On account of the nature of the topic, non-probability sampling techniques have been used. Despite best efforts to get a representative sample and remove personal biases, the study could be subject to limitations associated with such sampling techniques.
- On account of the sampling techniques adopted, non-parametric tools were used for analysis on account of their 'superior' nature; the same are, however, of *indicative* value only for others.

Glossary

Borrowings: These are all those borrowings, financial in nature, which the respondents have made or admitted of making for various reasons. These borrowings are either from banks, money lenders, employer, friends, neighbours, relatives or others; and are to be compulsorily repaid either with or without interest payment depending upon the source. For the purpose of this study, borrowings also include advances taken from the employer which are to be adjusted/debited from future salary/wage earnings. (See also *UUI*.)

Caregiver (CG): Person who takes care of an HIV+ sick individual. For the present study caregiving may be full time or part time.

Continuously: With reference to NHIEs, it refers to a member being regularly ill; such a member falls/is sick almost every single/ alternate day. (See also *frequently*.)

Dependants: Any non-earning member of any age group. As opposed to this, a working member is one who has a regular or full-time job: permanent, contractual or on day-to-day basis. Daily wage-earners who are capable of working and have been currently working, but whose job on a day-to-day basis is not guaranteed because of the very nature of such employment are not considered as dependants.

Dissavings: A term used to denote generation of resources to meet HH expenses wherein the concerned HH sells/liquidates assets/ past savings (for example, premature closure of term deposits).

Frequently: With reference to NHIEs, it refers to a member being ill 4–5 times a month or more; such a member falls/is sick about once a week. (See also *continuously*.)

Fully sponsored food: A term coined for the present study, it refers to food which is provided free to a HH throughout the month by an individual, institution or another HH. Here the HH under consideration does not spend any money on food. (See also *partly sponsored food* and *own food*.)

HIV/AIDS household: Refers to a HH where there is at least one living member in the age group of 18–60 years who is HIV+. (See also *non-HIV/AIDS household*.)

Hospitalized illness episode (HIE): Any illness episode which required at least one night or 24-hour stay either at a hospital or C&S Home. (See also *non-hospitalized illness episode*.)

Household (HH): Residential premise, abode or dwelling where members of a family are living, eating and staying together. Also, while a common entrance to the abode is made use of by all members, meals are cooked at one place and consumed by all members as a unit. Members of a HH comprise primarily the following: all those who stay together and are present in the dwelling; members who work elsewhere but return back regularly/periodically and contribute regularly to HH expenses; minors who may be in hostels or boarding schools. Adult family members who stay separate for reasons including settlement, marriage or work, and do not contribute in any way to the said HH are not part of the HH for the purpose of this study. A HH can also comprise a single member, who stays alone either due to eviction, ex-communication, and/or death/marriage of other members. A HH for the purpose of this study does not include unrelated individuals who for the purpose of employment or convenience stay together on an equal-cost-sharing basis. A dwelling having members belonging to the same family, staying under the same roof, but who make use of separate entrances and/or cook/eat separately is not considered as one HH. Such a place constitutes two separate HHs.

Household head: Generally, though not always, the senior most member in the HH in terms of age. The HH head is a person who is recognized as such by the HH. She or he is generally the person who bears the chief responsibility for managing the affairs of the

HH and takes decision on behalf of the HH. The definition is quite similar to the one of Census of India.

Household land: Refers to any land, plot or open space owned by the HH but not including the land on which the dwelling is on.

Literate member: A member who can read, write and understand basics of any language. For the purpose of the present study, a member is also considered as a literate member if he or she currently goes to school and is at least in Class I and above.

Minor: Any HH member who is below 18 years of age.

Non-HIV/AIDS household: HH without any HIV+ tested member. (See also *HIV/AIDS HH.*)

Non-hospitalized illness episode (NHIE): Any illness episode which requires medical attention, but which does not require hospitalization. (See also *hospitalized illness episode.*)

Non-wage income: Refers primarily to income from rent, dividends, pension, regular financial help from charitable organizations, etc. For the purpose of the present study, non-wage income is that which is not earned through direct, active, productive or gainful employment during the last one year. (See also *wage income.*)

Other annual household consumption expenditure: They are expenses which are not incurred regularly on a daily or monthly basis. While examples include expenses on medical treatment, education, repair/maintenance of house/vehicle, purchase of clothing/footwear, durable/electronic/electrical goods, etc.; daily food and regular monthly expenses on house-rent, electricity/water/fuel, phone, entertainment, TV, alcohol, toiletries, etc., are not part of the same.

Own food: A term coined for the present study, it refers to food which is entirely purchased with own funds by the HHs. (See also *fully sponsored food* and *partly sponsored food.*)

Partly sponsored food: This is another term coined exclusively for the present study. Besides the amount actually spent by the HH on food, an additional amount towards food is received by the

HH every month in cash or kind from external sources including NGOs. Actual food expenses of the HH thus stand reduced due to this assistance, if any. Also, besides HHs as a whole getting this support, certain categories of workers such as housemaids or those working in hotels/restaurants get part of their food requirements at the place of work on a daily basis, thus reducing their monthly HH food expenses. Partly sponsored food can also refer to the fact that of the actual food expenses shown, a part is reimbursed later by others such as relations. (See also *fully sponsored food* and *own food*.)

Total annual household income (or Total HH income): It is the sum of wage and non-wage income. It is approximate net income after taxes, if any, and after taking into consideration loss of income due to the absence of work on account of sickness and/ or caregiving. The total HH income is calculated inclusive of increments and bonuses, if any, and in case of wage earners by considering annual wages in approximate terms keeping in mind the feedback obtained from the respondent and other HH members (if any) and the average number of days the respondent went to work during the previous month.

Unrequited and/or unrevealed income (UUI): A term coined exclusively for the present study to define income (over and above borrowings) used by HHs to tide over deficits. If one does not consider this income, sources of which are often undisclosed, there can be no plausible explanation of how certain HHs cope with their deficits. UUI often comes from sources which are not revealed either initially or acknowledged even subsequently by the respondents. UUI is different from borrowings: while borrowings are acknowledged and verifiable, UUIs are often unverifiable and hidden, and could even be from dubious sources such as prostitution, gambling and petty crime/illegalities. UUI includes the following modes of getting funds: borrowing from close relatives/friends wherein the amount borrowed does not have to be returned (these are not considered by many as borrowings since they do not have to be returned; such a source of covering deficits is present across all income brackets particularly among the relatively better-off HHs; UUI of this form occur usually when on account of the adversity faced, a relatively better-off sibling or close relative provides some lump sum amount periodically or takes regular care of reimbursing pre-decided bills such as those pertaining to medicines, electricity, fuel, education, etc.); amount obtained from dubious sources/activities such as theft, prostitution and/or gambling (these sources of income or modes of covering deficits are usually concealed; their size cannot be minutely verified; that such modes exist have been confirmed by field workers/ NGOs; this is an important source/mode of additional income for some, especially from the lower income brackets, since these neither have assets for sale/liquidation to generate resources or to provide as security for borrowing, nor do they have rich relations who could assist on a regular basis on account of their own poor status.); amount received from foreign benefactors, NGOs, religious organizations, etc. (See also *borrowings*.)

Wage income: Refers primarily to income in the form of salary, wages, fees, commission, agricultural income, etc. Amongst others, it is income earned during the last year from direct employment, self-employment, business and trade. (See also *non-wage income*.)

References

ADB. 2004. *Asia's economies and the challenge of AIDS*. Asian Development Bank. Available online at http://www.adb.org/Documents/Books/Asia-AIDS/ (accessed July 2008).

ADB/UNAIDS. 2004. *Asia-Pacific's opportunity: Investing to avert an HIV/AIDS crisis*. ADB/UNAIDS Study Series. Bangkok and Manila: ADB/UNAIDS.

Adeyi, O., R. Hecht, E. Njobvu and A. Soucat. 2001. *AIDS, poverty reduction and debt relief: A toolkit for mainstreaming HIV/AIDS programmes into development instruments*. Geneva: UNAIDS/World Bank.

Ahiraj, M. 2007. Scheme to help bring smiles on the faces of HIV-affected. *The Hindu*, Karnataka, 12 October.

Ainsworth, Martha and Deon Filmer. 2002. 'Poverty, AIDS and children's schooling: A targeting dilemma', Policy Research Working Paper No. 2885, Washington: World Bank.

Albert, Terry and Gregory Williams. 1998. 'The economic burden of HIV/AIDS in Canada', CPRN Study No. H | 02 | (with collaboration of Barbara Legowski and Robert Remis), Ottawa: Renouf Publishing Co. Ltd. Available online at http://www.cprn.com/documents/18422_en.pdf (accessed August 2008).

Aliber, Michael, C. Walker, M. Machera, P. Kamau, C. Omondi and K. Kanyinga. 2004. 'The impact of HIV/AIDS on land rights: Case studies from Kenya.' Cape Town, South Africa: HSRC Publishers. Available online at http://www.fao.org/sd/dim_pe3/docs/pe3_040902d1_en.pdf (accessed May 2010).

Arndt, Channing and Jeffrey D. Lewis. 2000. 'The macro implications of HIV/AIDS in South Africa', Africa Region Working Paper Series, No. 9, Washington, DC: The World Bank.

Avert. 2008. 'Impact of HIV & AIDS in Africa'. Available online at http://www.avert.org/aidsimpact.htm (accessed May 2008).

Barnett, Tony and Alan Whiteside. 2000. *Guidelines for studies of the social and economic impact of HIV/AIDS*. Geneva, Switzerland: UNAIDS.

Barnett, T. and P. Blaikie. 1992. *AIDS in Africa: Its present and future impact*. New York: The Guilford Press.

Basu, Alaka, Deendra Gupta and Geetanjali Krishna. 1997. 'The households impact of adult morbidity and mortality: Some implications of the potential epidemics of AIDS in India', in David Bloom and Peter Goodwin (eds.), *The economics of HIV/AIDS: The case of South and South-east Asia*, pp. 102–154. New Delhi: Oxford University Press.

Bechu, N. 1998. 'The impact of AIDS on the economy of families of Cote d'Ivoire: Changes in consumption among AIDS affected households', in M. Ainsworth,

L. Fransen and M. Over (eds.), *Confronting AIDS: Evidence from the developing world*. Washington, DC: The World Bank.

Beegle, K. 2003. 'Labor effects of adult morality in Tanzanian households', Policy Research Working Paper No. 3062. Washington, DC: The World Bank.

Bell, Clive, Shantayanan Devarajan and Hans Gersbach. 2003. 'The long-run economic costs of AIDS: Theory and an application to South Africa', WPS3152. Washington DC: The World Bank.

————. 2004. 'Thinking about the long-run economic costs of AIDS', in Markus Haacker (ed.), *The macroeconomics of HIV/AIDS*, pp. 96–133. Washington DC: International Monetary Fund. Available online at http://www.imf.org/external/pubs/ft/AIDS/eng/ (accessed July 2008).

Beni, Romanus. 2008. 'The vulnerability of women to HIV/AIDS in Indonesia', in K. Prasad and U.V. Somayajulu (eds.), *HIV and AIDS vulnerability of women in Asia and Africa*, chap. 9, pp. 245–293. New Delhi: The Women Press.

Bertozzi, Stefano, Marjorie Opuni and Juan-Pablo Gutiérrez. 2001. 'The economic impacts of HIV/AIDS.' Available online at http://ipsnews.net/aids/page_5.shtml (accessed May 2010).

Bils, M. and P. Klenow. 2000. 'Does schooling cause growth?' *American Economic Review*, 90(5): 1160–1183.

Bisserbe, N. 2008. 'Corporate India wakes up to health risks', *The Economic Times*, Mumbai, 12 February.

Bloom, David E., David Canning and Pia Malaney. 2000. 'Demographic change and economic growth in East Asia', *Population and Development Review*, 26: 257–290.

Bloom, David, David Canning and Jaypee Sevilla. 2004. 'The effect of health on economic growth: A production function approach', *World Development*, January, pp. 1–13.

Bloom, David and Sherry Glied. 1993. 'Economic implications of AIDS in Asia', in David Bloom and Joyce Lyons (eds.), *Economic implications of AIDS in Asia*, New Delhi: Oxford University Press.

Bloom, David and Ajay Mahal. 1996. 'Economic implications of AIDS in Asia,' *Draft*. New York: Columbia University, Department of Economics.

————. 1997. 'AIDS, flu and black death' in D. Bloom and P. Godwin (eds.), *The economics of HIV and AIDS: The case of South and South-East Asia*, Godwin. Delhi: Oxford University Press.

Bloom, David E., River Path Associates and Jaypee Sevilla. 2001a. 'HIV/AIDS and development in Asia and the Pacific: A lengthening shadow – Health, wealth, AIDS and poverty.' Asia Pacific Ministerial Meeting, 9–10 October. Melbourne, Australia: The Australian Government's Overseas Aid Program. Available online at http://www.ausaid.gov.au/publications/pdf/health_wealth_poverty.pdf (accessed September 2008)

————. 2001b. 'Health, wealth, AIDS and poverty: The case of Cambodia.' Available online at http://www.iaen.org/files.cgi/7054_bloom_cambodia.pdf

Bloom, D. and J. Williamson. 1998. 'Demographic transitions and economic miracles in emerging Asia.' *World Bank Economic Review*, 12: 419–55.

Bollinger, L., J. Stover and P. Riwa. 1999. 'The economic impact of AIDS in Tanzania', Policy Working Paper. Policy Project. Available online at http://www.policyproject.com/pubs/SEImpact/tanzania.pdf (accessed February 2012)

Booysen, Frederick le Roux. 2003. 'Poverty dynamics and HIV/AIDS related morbidity and mortality in South Africa', Conference paper presented at

Empirical evidence for the demographic and socio-economic impact of AIDS. University of KwaZulu-Natal, March 26–28.

Booysen, Frikkie, Dingie van Rensburg, M. Bachmann, M. Engelbrecht and F. Steyn. 2002. 'The socioeconomic impact of HIV/AIDS on households in South Africa', *AIDS Bulletin:* 11(1).

Bora, Nitin. 2008. 'There is more to health than AIDS' in Rohini Sahni, V. Kalyan Shankar, and Hemant Apte (eds.), *Prostitution and Beyond*, chap. 19, pp. 268–275. New Delhi: SAGE Publications.

Canning, David, Ajay Mahal, Kunle Odumosu and Prosper Okonkwo. 2006a. 'Assessing the economic impact of HIV/AIDS on Nigerian households: A propensity score matching approach', Program on the Global Demography of Aging, Working Paper Series No. 16. Harvard Institute for Global Health. Available online at http://www.hsph.harvard.edu/pgda/working.htm (accessed September 2008).

———. 2006b. 'The economic impact of HIV/AIDS on Nigerian firms', in Olusoji Oadeyi, Phyllis Kanki, Oluwole Odutolu, and John Idoko (eds.), *AIDS in Nigeria: A nation on the threshold*, Cambridge MA: Harvard Center for Population and Development Studies.

Case, Anne, Christina H. Paxson and Joseph D. Ableidinger. 2004. 'Orphans in Africa: Parental death, poverty, and school enrollment', *Demography*, 41(3), August 2004: 483–508.

CEC (Centre for Education and Communication). 2004. 'HIV/AIDS.' Available online at http://www.cec-india.org/leftlinks/05/folder.2004-08-20.1290171887 (accessed June 2007).

Census of India. 2001. Table H-4 (Appendix) India. Available online at http://www.censusindia.gov.in/Census_Data_2001/States_at_glance/State_Links/30_goa.pdf (accessed November 2009).

Chatterjee, Ashoke and Kusum Sahgal. 2002. 'HIV/AIDS awareness and control: The role of non-governmental organizations in the country', in Samiran Panda, Anindya Chatterjee and Abu S. Abdul-Quader (eds.), *Living with the AIDS virus: The epidemic and the response in India*, chap. 3, pp. 62–76. New Delhi: SAGE Publications.

Chopra, Sanjeev. 2008. 'Rehabilitated? Not quite. An HIV+ve widow speaks out.' *The Indian Express*, Mumbai, 19 February.

Correa, Mariette and David Gisselquist. 2005. 'HIV from blood exposures in India – an exploratory study', Norwegian Church Aid (NCA), Regional Representation, South Asia.

Correa, Mariette, David Gisselquist and D.H. Gore. 2008. *Blood-borne HIV: Risks and prevention*. Chennai: Orient Longman.

Cuddington, J.T. 1993. 'Further results on the macroeconomic effects of AIDS: The dualistic labor-surplus economy', *World Bank Economic Review*. 7(3), May 1993: 403–417.

D'Cruz, Premilla. 2001. 'Children with HIV/AIDS: Beyond infected and affected', Paper prepared for UNICEF on behalf of Committed Communities Development Trust, Mumbai.

———. 2004. *Family care in HIV/AIDS: Exploring lived experience*. New Delhi: SAGE Publications.

Dhar, Aarti. 2007. 'HIV prevalence rate 0.28 p.c.: Survey', *The Hindu*, Karnataka, 10 October.

214   Economic Impact of HIV/AIDS on Households

Dixit, A.P. (ed.) 2005. *Global HIV/AIDS trends*. Delhi: Vista International Publishing House.
Dixon, Simon, S. McDonald and Jennifer Roberts. 2001. AIDS/HIV and development in Africa. *Journal of International Development*, 13(4): 411–426.
Donovan, Cynthia, Linda Bailey, Edson Mpyisi and Michael Weber. 2003. *Prime age adult morbidity and mortality in rural Rwanda: Effects on household income, agricultural production and food security strategies*. Kigali, Rwanda: Ministry of Agriculture, Livestock and Forestry.
Drummond, Don and Richard Kelly. 2006. 'The economic cost of AIDS: A clear case for action. *TD Economics – Special Report*; TD Bank Financial Group.' Available online at www.td.com/economics (accessed June 2008).
Duraisamy, Palanigounder. 2003. 'Economic impact of HIV/AIDS on patients and households in south India', presented at 11th IAEN Face-to-Face Conference. Available online at http://www.iaen.org/papers (accessed May 2005).
Duraisamy, P. C., R. Daly, A. Homan, N. Ganesh, A. Kumarasamy, P. Karim, Sri Priya, C. Castle, P. Verma, V. Mahendra and S. Solomon. 2003. 'The economic impact of HIV/AIDS in patients and households in South India', *Draft*. Chennai: University of Madras, Department of Econometrics.
Esparza, Jose and Saladin Osmanov. 2004. 'Current issues in HIV vaccine development' in J.P. Narain (ed.), *AIDS in Asia*, chap. 22, pp. 349–359. New Delhi: SAGE Publications.
Evans, David and Edward Miguel. 2004. 'Orphans and schooling in Africa: A longitudinal analysis', BREAD Working Paper No. 056, March 2004.
Falleiro, Savio. 2009. 'A study of HIV/AIDS awareness among college students in Goa vis-à-vis their socio-economic profile', Minor Research Project under the assistance of University Grants Commission.
———. 2010. 'Sex education in the times of HIV/AIDS', *Goa Today*, 45(1): 72–74.
Falleiro, Savio and S. Noronha. 2011. 'Newer perspectives on the burden of HIV/AIDS on medical expenditures on individuals and households', *Journal of Health Management*, 13(3): 301–328.
———. 2012. 'Economic impact of HIV/AIDSA on women', *Journal of Health Management*, 14(4): 495–512.
FAO. 2004. 'HIV/AIDS, gender inequality and rural livelihoods: The impact of HIV/AIDS on rural livelihoods in Northern Province, Zambia, Rome, Food and Agriculture Organization, Development Cooperation Ireland (DCI), Government of Zambia.' Available online at http://www.fao.org/sd/dim_pe1/pe1_040602_en.htm (accessed September 2008).
Farmer, Paul. 1999. *Infections and Inequalities*. University of California Press.
Ferreira, Pedro C. and Samuel D. Pessoa. 2003. 'The long-run economic impact of AIDS', Working Paper (10 February 2003). Available online at http://papers.ssrn.com/sol3/papers.cfm?abstract_id=411782. (abstract accessed September 2008)
Foulkes, Imogen. 2008. 'Aids epidemic - a global disaster.' Available online at http://news.bbc.co.uk/2/hi/health/7474600.stm (accessed June 2008).
Fox, M.P., J.L. Simon, M. Bii, K.M. Wasunna, W.B. MacLeod, G. Foglia and S. Rosen. 2003. 'The impact of HIV/AIDS on labour productivity in Kenya', Paper Presented at the Scientific Meeting on Empirical Evidence for the Demographic and Socio-economic Impact of AIDS, hosted by the Health Economics and HIV/AIDS Research Division (HEARD), Durban, 26–28 March.

Fox, M.P, Sydney Rosen, William B. MacLeod, Monique Wasunna, Margaret Bii, Ginamarie Foglia and Jonathon L. Simon. 2004. 'The impact of HIV/AIDS on labour productivity in Kenya', *Tropical Medicine and International Health*, 9(3): 318–324. Available online at http://info.worldbank.org/etools/library/latestversion.asp?135887 (accessed September 2008).

Fredricksson, Jenni and Annabel Kanabus. 2007. 'The impact of HIV & AIDS on Africa.' Available online at http://www.avert.org/aidsimpact.htm (accessed July 2007).

Gaigbe-Togbe, Victor and Mary Beth Weinberger. 2003. 'The social and economic implications of HIV/AIDS. *African Population Studies Supplement B to vol 19; United Nations - New York: Population Division, Department of Economic and Social Affairs.'* Available online at https://tspace.library.utoronto.ca/bitstream/1807/5825/1/ep04034.pdf (accessed August 2008).

Gaitonde, I.R. 2001. *A Thief in the Night: Understanding AIDS*. Chennai: East West Books.

Garg, Abhinav. 2010. 'Pregnancy care denied, HC orders relief.', *The Times of India*, Goa, 07 June.

Gautham, Meenakshi. 2008. 'Hope after HIV.', *The Hindu magazine*, 30 November. Available online at http://www.hindu.com/mag/2008/11/30/stories/2008113050010100.htm (accessed March 2011).

Government of Goa. *Economic Survey, 2005–2006*. Government of Goa.

Greener, Robert. 2004. 'The impact of HIV on poverty and inequality', in Markus Haacker (ed.), *The macroeconomics of AIDS and poverty*, Washington DC: IMF.

GSACS. 2005–2006. 'HIV/AIDS in Goa: Situation and response'. Goa State AIDS Control Society, Panaji.

———. 2008. 'HIV/AIDS in Goa: Situation and response'. Goa State AIDS Control Society, Panaji.

———. 2009. 'HIV/AIDS in Goa: Situation and response'. Goa State AIDS Control Society, Panaji. Available online at http://goasacs.nic.in/hivaidsingoa2009.pdf (accessed May 2010).

———. 2010. 'HIV/AIDS in Goa.', Goa State AIDS Control Society. Panaji. Available online at http://goasacs.nic.in/goa-HIV-data2010.pdf (accessed March 2013).

Gupta, I. 1998. 'Planning for the socio-economic impact of the epidemic: The costs of being ill.', in P. Godwin (ed.), *The looming epidemic: The impact of HIV/AIDS in India*. Delhi: Mosaic Books.

Gupta, Indrani and Samiran Panda. 2002. 'The HIV/AIDS epidemic in India: Looking ahead', in Samiran Panda, A. Chatterjee and Abu S. Abdul-Quader (eds.), *Living with the AIDS virus: The epidemic and the response in India*, chap. 10, pp. 179–196. New Delhi: SAGE Publications.

Gupta, Indrani, Mayur Trivedi and Subodh Kandamuthan. 2007. *Adoption of health technologies in India: Implications for the AIDS vaccine*. New Delhi: SAGE Publications.

Hosegood, Victoria, Kobus Herbst and Ian Timæus. 2003. 'The impact of adult AIDS deaths on households and children's living arrangements in rural South Africa.', Paper presented at the scientific meeting on Empirical Evidence for the Demographic and Socio-economic Impact of AIDS, hosted by the Health Economics and HIV/AIDS Research Division (HEARD), Durban, March 26–28.

Hosegood et al. 2004. 'The impact of adult mortality on household dissolution and migration in rural South Africa', *AIDS*, 23, 18 (11), July 23.

HRLN. 2008. 'A judicial colloquium – HIV / AIDS and the law'. Human Rights Law Network, New Delhi.

ILO. 2003. 'Socio-economic impact of HIV / AIDS on people living with HIV / AIDS and their families', ILO India Project: Prevention of HIV / AIDS in the world of work: A tripartite response. *ILO Publications*, New Delhi.

IMF. 2005. 'The IMF's role in the fight against HIV / AIDS: A factsheet – September 2005'. Available online at http://www.imf.org/external/np/exr/facts/mdg.htm (accessed February 2008).

Israni, A.S. 2001. 'HIV / AIDS and STD: An information manual. New Delhi: *Commonwealth Publishers*.

Jacob, K.S. 2007. 'Errors of the public health movement'. *The Hindu*, 6 December.

Jain, Dipika. 2008a. 'Against mandatory pre-marital HIV testing in India'. Human Rights Law Network, New Delhi.

Jain, Dipika and Rachel Stephens. 2008. 'The struggle for access to treatment for HIV / AIDS in India'. Human Rights Law Network, New Delhi.

Jain, Sonu. 2008b. 'AIDS programme infected: Bribes for contracts, dubious NGOs, political strings'. *The Indian Express*, 16 January.

Joshi, P.L. 2000. 'HIV / AIDS in India', in Sushma Gupta and O.P. Sood (eds.), *HIV/ AIDS in India*, 6(5): 27–32, Proceedings of the Sixth Round Table Conference, Round Table Conference Series, Ranbaxy Science Foundation, New Delhi, 5 April.

Kabir, M. 2008. 'Sexually transmitted infections and HIV/AIDS vulnerability in Bangladesh', in K. Prasad and U.V. Somayajulu (eds.), *HIV and AIDS vulnerability of women in Asia and Africa*, chap 7, pp. 182–216. New Delhi: The Women Press.

Kadiyala, Suneetha and Tony Barnett. 2004. 'AIDS in India: Disaster in the making'. *Economic and Political Weekly*, 8 May: 1888–1892.

Kakar, D.N., and S.N. Kakar. 2001. *Combating AIDS in the 21st century: Issues and challenges*. New Delhi: Sterling Publishers Private Limited.

Kelly, B., B. Raphael, D. Statham, M. Ross, H. Eastwood, S.O. Mclean, et al. 1996. 'A comparison of psychosocial aspects of AIDS and cancer related bereavement.' *Int J Psychiatr Med*, 26: 35–49.

KFF (Henry J. Kaiser Family Foundation). 2002. Available online at *Hitting home: How households cope with the impact of the HIV/AIDS epidemic*. http://www.kff.org/southafrica/20021125a-index.cfm (accessed October 2008).

Kinnon, Colette M., German Velasquez and Yves-Antoine Flori. 1994. *Health economics: A guide to selected WHO literature*. WHO Task Force on Health Economics.

Krishnamoorthy, E.S. 2009. 'Quest for the ideal healthcare model'. *The Hindu*, 4 November.

———. 2010. 'At healthcare's fountainhead'. *The Hindu*, 5 May.

Mahal, Ajay, and Bhargavi Rao. 2005. 'HIV / AIDS epidemic in India: An economic perspective'. *Indian J Med Res*, 121, April: 582–600.

Mahal, A. and M. Seshu. 2000. *Social security among sex workers in Sangli*. Sangli, India: Sampada Grameen Mahila Sanstha (SANGRAM).

Mahapatra, Dhananjay. 2008. 'BPL status for AIDS patients'. *The Times of India*, 6 August.

———. 2010. 'AIDS control budget slashed'. *The Times of India*, 17 September.

Mascarenhas, Anuradha. 2006. 'Blood bonds'. *The Sunday Express*, 14 May.

Mawar, N. and R.S. Paranjape. 2002. 'Live and let live: Acceptance of people living with HIV/AIDS in an era where stigma and discrimination persist'. *ICMR Bull*, 32: 105–114.

Mawar, Nita, Seema Sahay, Apoorvaa Pandit, and Uma Mahajan. 2005. 'The third phase of HIV pandemic: Social consequences of HIV/AIDS stigma & discrimination & future needs'. *Indian J Med Res*, 122, December: 471–484.

McGuire, Alistair, John Henderson and Gavin Mooney. 1997. *The economics of health care*. London: Routledge.

Medhini, Laya, Dipika Jain and Colin Gonsalves (eds.) 2007a. *HIV/AIDS and the law – Volume I*. New Delhi: HRLN.

———. 2007b. *HIV/AIDS and the law – Volume II*. New Delhi: HRLN.

Mehdi, Ali. 2008. 'Is curative care the cure?' *The Economic Times*, 9 February.

Misra, Geetanjali, A. Mahal and R. Shah. 2008. 'Protecting the rights of sex workers: The Indian experience', in G. Misra and R. Chandiramani (eds.), *Sexuality, gender and rights: Exploring theory and practice in South and Southeast Asia*, chap.12, pp. 219–242. New Delhi: SAGE Publications.

Mohanty, Hrusikesh. 2008. 'Orissa to pay ₹200 as pension to HIV+'. *The Times of India*, 8 February.

Nagarajan, Rema. 2007. 'HIV+ most ostracized by doctors'. *The Times of India*, 27 December.

Nagarsekar, Rajeshree. 2009. 'GSACS ropes in 3 clinics to provide free HIV testing'. *The Times of India*, 1 December.

Nair, P. 2008a. 'Desperate acts by Goa's HIV+ve'. *The Times of India*, 11 June.

———. 2008b. 'Free drugs for AIDS patients'. *The Times of India*, 07 June.

———. 2009a. 'Sex workers in Goa more likely to end life'. *The Times of India*, 4 June.

———. 2009b. 'No toast to your good health, this'. *The Times of India*, 24 January.

———. 2009c. 'Only 39% aware of HIV prevention'. *The Times of India*, 8 May.

Nampanya-Serpell, Namposya. 2000. 'Social and economic risk factors for HIV/AIDS affected families in Zambia'. Paper presented at the AIDS and Economics Symposium, Durban South Africa, 7–8 July.

Narain, Jai, P. 2004. 'AIDS in Asia: The epidemic profile and lessons learnt so far', in Jai. P. Narain (ed.), *AIDS in Asia: The challenge ahead*, chap. 1, pp.19–41. New Delhi: WHO and SAGE Publications.

Narain, Jai P and Charles F. Gilks. 2004. 'The "3 by 5" initiative: Challenges and opportunities for Asia', in Jai P. Narain (ed.), *AIDS in Asia: The challenge ahead*, chap. 6, pp. 107–121. New Delhi: WHO and SAGE Publications.

NCAER. 2004. *Socio-economic impact study of HIV/AIDS: Questionnaire for HIV/AIDS households*. New Delhi: National Council for Applied Economic Research.

Neuman, W. Lawrence. 2000. *Social Research Methods: Qualitative and Quantitative Approaches*. Boston: Allyn and Bacon.

Nielsen, Jette and Bjorn Melgaard. 2004. 'The economic and security dimensions of HIV/AIDS in Asia', in Jai P. Narain (ed.), *AIDS in Asia: The challenge ahead*, chap. 2, pp. 42–57. New Delhi: WHO and SAGE Publications.

Ojha, Vijay P., and Basanta K. Pradhan. 2006. *The macro-economic and sectoral impacts of HIV and AIDS in India: A CGE analysis*. New Delhi: UNDP.

Over, Mead. 1992. The macroeconomic impact of AIDS in Sub-Saharan Africa. Mimeo. Washington DC: The World Bank.

———. 2004. 'Impact of the HIV/AIDS epidemic on the health sectors of developing countries', in Markus Haacker (ed.), *The macro economics of HIV/AIDS*, chap. 10, pp. 311–344. International Monetary Fund. Available online at http://www. imf.org/external/pubs/ft/AIDS/eng/ (accessed July 2010).

Over, M., P. Heywood, J. Gold, I. Gupta, S. Hira and E. Marseille. 2004. *HIV/AIDS treatment and prevention in India: Modeling the costs and consequences*. Washington, D.C.: The World Bank.

Panagariya, Arvind. 2008. 'The crisis in rural health care'. *The Economic Times*, 24 January.

Panda, P.K., A. Bhoi, Y. Singh and K. Sankaraiyah. 2007. 'Health status of tribals in India: Evidence from Andhra Pradesh', in Himanshu Sekhar Rout and P.K. Panda (eds.), *Health Economics in India*, chap. 5, pp. 67–79. New Delhi: New Century Publications.

Panda, Samiran, Anindya Chatterjee and Abu S. Abdul-Quader, eds. 2002. *Living with the AIDS virus: The epidemic and the response in India*. New Delhi: SAGE Publications.

Pande, J.N. 2000. 'National approaches to AIDS disease management', in Sushma Gupta and O.P. Sood (eds.), *HIV/AIDS in India*, 6(12): 113–120, Proceedings of the Sixth Round Table Conference, Round Table Conference Series, Ranbaxy Science Foundation, New Delhi, 5 April.

Pandey, Shruti. 2006. 'Fight for free ARV drugs'. *Combat Law*, April–May: 5(2).

Pavri, Khorshed M. 1996. *Challenge of AIDS*. New Delhi: National Book Trust.

Pereira, A. 2008. 'How HIV has now become a lifestyle disease'. *The Times of India*, 24 May.

Pitayanon, Sumalee, Sukontha Kongsin and Wattana Janjaeron, 1997. 'The economic impact of HIV/AIDS mortality on households in Thailand', in David Bloom and Peter Godwin (eds.), *The economics of HIV and AIDS: The case of South and Southeast Asia*, pp. 53–101. New Delhi: Oxford University Press.

Pradhan, Basanta K. and Ramamani Sundar. 2006. 'Gender impact of HIV and Aids in India'. New Delhi: NCAER, NACO and UNDP.

Pradhan, Basanta K., Ramamani Sundar and Shalabh K. Singh. 2006. 'Socio-economic impact of HIV and AIDS in India'. New Delhi: NCAER, NACO and UNDP. Also available at: http://data.undp.org.in/hivreport/India_Report.pdf (assessed on October 2009).

Prasad, Kiran. 2008. 'Women's vulnerability to HIV/AIDS in Asia and Africa', in Kiran Prasad and U.V. Somayajulu (eds.), *HIV and AIDS vulnerability of women in Asia and Africa*, chap.1, pp. 1–57. New Delhi: The Women Press.

Prasad, Kiran and U.V. Somayajulu (eds.). 2008. 'HIV and AIDS vulnerability of women in Asia and Africa'. New Delhi: The Women Press.

Punnyakamo, Sommai. 2001. 'Coming to terms with truth'. *Choices*, 10(4).

Rajadhyaksha, M. 2009. 'New health bill boosts patient's rights'. *The Times of India*, 2 February.

Ramachandran, R. and T.K. Rajalakshmi. 2009. 'Unhealthy trend'. *Frontline*, 10 April: 21–25.

Ramaiah, Savitri (ed.). 2008. *Health solutions: HIV/AIDS*. New Delhi: Sterling Paperbacks.

Ramakrishna, Jayashree, P.J. Pelto, R.K. Verma, S.L. Schensul and A. Joshi. 2008. 'Guidelines for policy-making and interventions in the time of AIDS', in R.K. Verma, P.J. Pelto, S.L. Schensul, and A. Joshi (eds.), *Sexuality in the time of AIDS: Contemporary perspectives from communities in India*, chap. 16, pp. 382–398. New Delhi: SAGE Publications.

Ramamurthy, V. 2004. *Strategic approaches to HIV and AIDS prevention and control.* New Delhi: Authors Press.

Ramani, K.V., Dileep Mavalankar and Dipti Govil (eds.). 2008. *Strategic issues and challenges in health management.* New Delhi: SAGE Publications.

Rao, Digumarti Bhaskara (ed.). 2000a. *HIV/AIDS: Issues and challenges – Part I.* New Delhi: Discovery Publishing House.

————. 2000b. *HIV/AIDS: Issues and Challenges – Part II.* New Delhi: Discovery Publishing House.

————. 2000c. *HIV/AIDS: Prevention education for educational institutions.* New Delhi: Discovery Publishing House.

Rao, Raghvendra. 2008. 'Rlys plans to go HIV+, may offer 75pc concession in fares to patients'. *The Indian Express,* 1 January.

Rashid, Toufiq. 2006. 'Four lakh AIDS deaths in India last year, highest in the world'. *The Indian Express,* 14 June.

Reddy, Vasudha. 2006. 'Tales of discrimination'. *Combat Law,* April–May, 5(2).

Reid, Elizabeth. 2000a. 'The HIV epidemic as a development issue', in Digumarti Bhaskara Rao (ed.), *HIV/AIDS: Issues and challenges – Part I,* chap. 3: 18–25. New Delhi: Discovery Publishing House.

————. 2000b. 'The HIV epidemic and development: The unfolding of the epidemic', in Digumarti Bhaskara Rao (ed.), *HIV/AIDS: Issues and challenges – Part I,* chap. 4, pp. 26–41. New Delhi: Discovery Publishing House.

————. 2000c. 'Challenges for UNDP in a changing world 1990-2000: Social trends', in Digumarti Bhaskara Rao (ed.), *HIV/AIDS: Issues and challenges – Part II,* chap. 47, pp. 778–785. New Delhi: Discovery Publishing House.

Roy, Debabrata (ed.). 2001. *Community action on HIV for Indian NGOs.* New Delhi: Voluntary Health Association of India (VHAI).

Sachs, Jeffrey D. 2008. 'Scaling up health in low income settings', in K.V. Ramani, Dileep Mavalankar and Dipti Govil (eds.), *Strategic issues and challenges in health management,* chap. 1, pp. 1–6. New Delhi: SAGE Publications.

Schoub, Barry D. 1995. *AIDS and HIV in perspective.* Great Britain: Cambridge University Press.

Sengupta, D. 2000. 'Clinical management of HIV/AIDS: Constraints', in Sushma Gupta and O.P. Sood (eds.), *HIV/AIDS in India,* 13(6): 121–126, Proceedings of the Sixth Round Table Conference, Round Table Conference Series, Ranbaxy Science Foundation, New Delhi, 5 April.

Sharma, Savita. 2006. *HIV/AIDS and You.* New Delhi: APH Publishing Corporation.

Sharma, S.N. and Amitabh Baxi. 2007. 'Crippling corporate'. *The Economic Times,* 12 August.

Shaukat, Mohammed and Salil Panakadan. 2004. 'HIV/AIDS in India: Problem and response', in Jai P. Narain (ed.), *AIDS in Asia: The challenge ahead,* Chap. 9, pp. 158–170. New Delhi: WHO and SAGE Publications.

Sheth, Parul R. 2004. *AIDS: A fatal gateway.* New Delhi: National Institute of Science Communication and Information Resources, CSIR.

Shrinivasan, Rukmini. 2010. 'A nation forced to go on distress diet'. *Sunday Times of India,* 1 August.

Singh, Anju (ed.). 2003. *What if everything you though you knew about AIDS was wrong?* (excerpts from Christine Maggiore's, 'What if everything you knew about AIDS was wrong?'). New Delhi: Polemics Communications.

220   Economic Impact of HIV/AIDS on Households

Singhal, Arvind and Everett M. Rogers. 2006. *Combating AIDS: Communication strategies in action*. New Delhi: SAGE Publications.
Sinha, K. 2006a. 'India home to 60% of S Asia's HIV patients'. *The Times of India*, 17 August.
——. 2006b. '38% of HIV-affected in India are women'. *The Times of India*, 23 November.
——. 2007. 'India third on AIDS list'. *The Times of India*, 8 July.
——. 2008. 'Over 2.1m kids under 15 in India living with HIV'. *The Times of India*, 5 April.
——. 2010a. 'Diabetes to bleed India of $32 this yr'. *The Times of India*, 11 August.
——. 2010b. '2.6L HIV patients have no access to treatment'. *The Times of India*, 1 October.
——. 2010c. 'Drug-resistant TB sweeps India: Report'. *Sunday Times of India*, 21 March.
Sinha, Sunita. 1995. *AIDS awareness*. New Delhi: Anmol Publications Pvt. Ltd.
Solomon, Suniti, Purnima Madhivanan, and A.K Ganesh. 2000. 'Mother to child transmission of HIV: Situation in India and programme implications'. in Sushma Gupta and O.P. Sood (eds.), *HIV/AIDS in India*, 6(10):99–105, Proceedings of the Sixth Round Table Conference, Round Table Conference Series, Ranbaxy Science Foundation, New Delhi, 5 April.
Thomas, Gracious, N.P. Sinha and J. Thomas K. 1997. *AIDS, Social Work and Law*. New Delhi: Rawat Publications.
UNAIDS. 2000a. 'AIDS epidemic update', December. Available online at http://www.unaids.org/wac/2000/wad00/files/WAD_epidemic_report_.htm
——. 2000b. 'Report on the Global HIV/AIDS epidemic', pp. 26–36, Geneva.
——. 2000c. 'Caring for carers'. Geneva: UNAIDS.
——. 2001. 'Investing in our future: Psychological support affected by HIV/AIDS'. Geneva: UNAIDS.
——. 2002. 'Report on the global AIDS epidemic'. New York.
——. 2006. 'Report on the global AIDS epidemic'. Geneva: UNAIDS. Available online at http://www.unaids.org/en/HIV_data/2006GlobalReport/default.asp (accessed August 2008)
——. 2008. 'Report on the global AIDS epidemic', Geneva: UNAIDS. Available online at http://www.unaids.org/en/KnowledgeCentre/HIVData/GlobalReport/2008/ (accessed August 2008).
——. 2010. 'Global report: UNAIDS report on the global AIDS epidemic 2010'. Available online at http://www.unaids.org/globalreport/Global_report.htm (accessed May 2012).
UNAIDS/UNICEF/USAID. 2002. 'Children on the brink 2002'. Washington DC: TvT.
UNDP. 2003. 'Regional human development report: HIV/AIDS and development in South Asia'.
UNDP. 2005. 'Human development report - International cooperation at a crossroads: Aid, trade and security in an unequal world'. New York. Available online at http://hdr.undp.org/reports/global/2005/(accessed August 2008).
UNESC/ESCAP. 2004. 'Selected issues in poverty reduction (item 8 of provisional agenda)', United Nations Economic and Social Council/Economic and Social Commission for Asia and the Pacific, Subcommittee on Poverty Reduction Practices, First session, 30 June–2 July, Bangkok.

UNFPA. 2005. 'State of the World Population 2005: Reproductive health - A measure of equity', chap. 4. Available online at http://www.unfa.org/swp/2005/english/chp4/chap4_page 1.htm (accessed November 2010).

Verma, Ravi and Tarun K. Roy. 2002. 'HIV risk behaviour and the sociocultural environment in India', in Samiran Panda, Anindya Chatterjee and Abu S. Abdul-Quader (eds.), *Living with the AIDS virus: The epidemic and the response in India*, chap 4, pp. 78–90. New Delhi: SAGE Publications.

Verma, Ravi K., S. Salil, Verra Mendonca, S.K. Singh, R. Prasad and R.B. Upadhyaya. 2002. 'HIV/AIDS and children in the Sangli District of Maharashtra (India)', in G.A. Cornia (ed.), *AIDS, public policy and child well-being*, New York/Nairobi: UNICEF.

Walker, A.J., C.C. Pratt and L. Eddy. 1995. 'Informal caregiving to aging family members'. *Family Relations*, 41: 402–41.

WCC. 2002. *Facing Aids* (A WCC Study Document), Geneva: WCC Publications.

Weil, D. 2001. *Accounting for the effect of health on economic growth*. Mimeo. Brown University.

Werker, Eric, Amrita Ahuja and Brian Wendell. 2007. 'Male circumcision and AIDS: The macroeconomic impact of a health crisis'. Working paper. USA (Harvard Business School/Lehman Brothers).

Whiteside, A. 2002. 'The economics of HIV/AIDS. *Plenary presentation at the International AIDS Economics of AIDS in Developing Countries Symposium*, Barcelona, 6 July'. Available online at http://www.iaen.org/files.cgi/7341_whiteside.pdf.

World Bank. 1997. 'Confronting AIDS: Public priorities in a global epidemic', A World Bank Policy Research Report, Oxford University Press.

———. 2000. 'HIV/AIDS in the Caribbean: Issues and Options—A background Report'. No. 20491-LAC, June.

———. 2003. 'World Development Report'. New York: Oxford University Press.

WHO. 1995. 'Global Programme on AIDS: 1992–1993 Progress Report'. Geneva: World Health Organization.

Xiaoge, Xu. 2008. 'AIDS, vulnerability of women and medical response in China', in K. Prasad and U.V. Somayajulu, *HIV and AIDS vulnerability of women in Asia and Africa*, chap. 8, pp. 217–243. New Delhi: The Women Press.

Yamano, Takashi and Thomas S. Jayne. 2004. 'Working-age adult mortality and primary school attendance in rural Kenya', Working Paper No. 005/2004, Tegemeo Institute of Agricultural Policy and Development.

Index

absenteeism, 10, 17, 31, 34, 36, 43, 46, 51, 159, 170, 177
Acquired Immunodeficiency Syndrome (AIDS)
cases reported/detected in Goa, 5–6
chronological stages in, 3
consequences of, 9
definition of, 1
economic impacts of, 171
epidemic in India, 2–3, 183
illness episodes, 138
medical care, 138
onset of, 145
'treatment' aspect of, 177
adherence, 161–162, 177–178
Adolescence Life Skills, 175
agricultural workers, HIV/AIDS impact on, 23, 28
AIDS Epidemic Update (2006), 2
Allied Insurance Company, 182
allopathic medicines, 160
market prices, 167n31
anti-retroviral (ARV) drugs, 11, 179
anti-retroviral treatment (ART), 66–67, 75, 120–122, 145–149, 168n35, 178
comparison with RMMT expenditure, 150
cost of, 177
expenses for, 148, 155
first-line treatment, 177
'Four Frees and One Care' programme, China, 183

highly active ART (HAART), 177
for HIV+ pregnant women, 176
link-ART centres, 177
second-line treatment, 177
Antyodaya Anna Yojana (AAY) scheme, 181
Apna Ghar (Goa), 182
Asia, 3, 173
assets, 28–29, 71–72, 91, 94, 97–98, 100–102, 106, 108, 115, 121, 161, 164, 172

bank loans, 180
Barre-Sinoussi, Francoise, 2
Behavioural Surveillance Survey, 174
Bellary District AIDS Prevention Society (BDAPS), 180
below poverty line (BPL), 178, 181–182. *See also* poverty line
bio-medical health, 179
blood banks, 176
blood product transmission, 7
blood supply, by licensed commercial banks, 176
blood transfusion, 176
budgets, of developing countries, 9

capital accumulation, 85, 120
care and support homes (C&S Homes), 126, 140, 145, 151, 155, 159–160, 163, 202–203

caregiving/caregivers (CGs), 37
  age of and amounts lost due to
    caregiving, 38
  amount lost per month, 41
  benefits of, 38
  caregivers currently not
    employed, 41
  identity, employment,
    occupation and age of, 39
  loss of employment and income,
    48–51
  need for, in the households, 38
  present and past employment
    status of, 199
CD-4 count test, 1, 66, 75, 146–149,
  162, 178
Center for Disease Control, 1
children's future, provision for,
  112–113
chi-square test, 203
chronic diseases, 11, 120, 145, 163
collateral, 101, 106
commercial sex workers (CSWs),
  8, 118n38
Commission on Macroeconomics
  and Health (CMH), 161, 174
Community Health Centres
  (CHC), 130
compensation, financial, 27, 43, 172
consumption expenses, of HIV/
  AIDS households, 68–75, 159
coping mechanisms, 65, 164
  adopted and total annual HH
    income slabs, 199
  adoption of, 47, 84, 170, 172
  pertaining to income and
    employment, 45–47
  used by HIV/AIDS HHs, 64
credit and social investment
  schemes, 180
'curative' measures, for HIV/
  AIDS infection
  'general curative' measures,
    180–183

'medico-curative' measures,
  176–179
curative medicine, 179

Dayanand Social Security Scheme
  (DSSS), 181
dead AIDS members, 23. *See also*
  HIV/AIDS member, death of
  age and employment of, 197–198
  details pertaining to, 21
death certificates, 6, 117n29
demographic
  demographic gift, 22
  reverse demographic gift, 22
denial of treatment, 168n37
dependence for assistance, modes
  of, 111–112
dependants, in HIV/AIDS HHs,
  16
Directorate of Women and Child
  Development, 182
disbanding, 16, 19
discrimination of people, suffering
  from HIV/AIDS, 32. *See also*
  people living with HIV/AIDS
  (PLWHA)
  at workplace, 182
dissavings, 61, 82, 88–89, 92, 94,
  98–100, 106–107, 141, 159, 164, 170
dissolution of HHs, 16, 19, 204
division of labour, 10
double employment and sources
  of income, loss of, 51–54
drug resistance, development of,
  161–162
drug users, 8

economic causes of HIV/AIDS,
  8, 13
economic costs of AIDS, 10, 22
economic empowerment, of HIV/
  AIDS victim, 180
economic hardships, of HIV/
  AIDS, 169

educational qualifications, of HH members, 14, 191–192, 201
educational system, impact of AIDS/HIV on, 78
Adolescence Life Skills, 175
educative programmes, adoption of, 176
importance of, 174
sex education, 175
women's education and, 174
Employee State Insurance Scheme (ESIS), 113
employment generation schemes, 180
employment of HIV+ respondents
'change in job' status, 25
coping mechanisms pertaining to, 45–47
double employment and sources of income, loss of, 51–54
in female-headed households, 46
financial compensation, 27
impact due to absenteeism caused by illness, 34–35
impact of HIV/AIDS on, 13–14
loss of, 23, 48–51
monthly income slabs, 30–31
present employment, 32–37
previous and present employment, 24–32
reasons for leaving job, 26
remunerative, 171
empowerment cost, 42
entrepreneurship programmes, home-based, 180
epidemics, 1–3, 7–10, 173, 180, 183
essential drugs, access to, 177

female-headed HHs, 23–24, 45–47, 52, 63–64, 75, 79, 81, 84, 86, 93, 98, 104, 113–114, 132, 171
annual non-wage income of, 18
borrowings in, 103

disadvantage of, 18, 68, 86, 113, 147
gender bias, 170
sponsored food for, 62
feminization of the epidemic, 7
Fisher's Exact Test, 203
Focus Group Discussion (FGD), 203
food assistance and security, 181
food expenses, of HIV/AIDS households, 60–68
association between gender and, 64
consumption of food, 61
dietary intake, 66
food-related hardships, 66
fully sponsored food, 62, 65
monthly expenses, 63–64
partly sponsored food, 61–62, 65–66
per capita expenditure, 61
ration-cards, 66
food inflation, 171
food insecurity, 67, 167n29
food insufficiency, 171
'Four Frees and One Care' programme, China, 183
fully sponsored food, 62–63, 65, 166n23, 171
funeral, 10, 23, 37, 44, 92

gay-related immunodeficiency (GRID), 2
gender biases, against females, 11, 178
gender inequalities, 8, 114, 180
Global Fund for Care, Support and Treatment (GFCST), 185n17
Goa Agriculture Department, 181
Goa State AIDS Control Society (GSACS), 5
Goa State Horticulture Corporation Limited (GSHCL), 181

government hospitals, 130, 140, 145, 151, 155, 163
gross domestic product (GDP), 9–10, 120
group insurance plan, 182

health care
  accessibility of, 121
  cost-effectiveness of, 172
  deficiency of public sector in, 161
  discrimination in, 163, 177
  essential drugs, access to, 177
  financial incapacity to pay, 163
  investment in, 176
  public health care, 178
health-related and medical
  expenses, of HIV/AIDS HHs, 60, 81, 146, 156–157, 170
  and accessibility of health care, 121
  allopathic medicines, 160
  annual expenditure, 122–126
  comparative profile of HHs, 123
  consultation fees and medicines, 133
  cost-effective strategy for, 174
  'free' government treatment, 155
  high treatment costs, 121
  hospitalized illness episodes/ treatment (HIEs/HIT), 136–145
  medical expense slabs, 125
  non-hospitalized illness episodes (NHIEs), 126–136
  non-hospitalized illness treatment (NHIT), 122, 126–136
  other annual HH consumption expenditure, 124
  private treatment, 133, 160–163
  Regular Monthly Medical Treatment (RMMT), 122, 145–155

health technologies, availability of, 176–177
highly active ART (HAART), 177
high-risk groups, 8, 175
HIV/AIDS member, death of, 19–24. *See also* dead AIDS members
  details pertaining to, 21
hospitalized illness episodes/ treatment (HIEs/HIT), 122, 136–145
  expense slabs of, 143
household expenditure
  categories of, 60
  on clothing/footwear, 81
  consumption expenditure, 68–75, 159
  and disproportionate burden on female members, 114–115
  on food, 60–68
  health-related and medical. *See* health-related and medical expenses, of HIV/AIDS HHs
  non-health consumption expenditure, 76
  other consumption expenditure, 76–84
  remittances, 84–85
  savings and investments, 85–89
household rupee, inflow of
  borrowings, 100–103
  versus unrequited and/or unrevealed income, 104–109
  dissavings, 98–100
  household income, 92–93
  others, 94–98
  total inflow, 109–111
  unrequited and/or unrevealed income, 103–104
household rupee, outflow of, 59
  household expenditure
    monthly expenditure on food, 60–68

monthly household
consumption expenditure,
68–75
other annual consumption
expenditure, 76–84
remittances, 84–85
savings and investments, 85–89
total outflow, 89–92
households, HIV/AIDS
children's future, provision for,
112–113
consumption expense slabs of,
76
dependence for assistance,
modes of, 111–112
economic impact of, 200
expenditure. *See* household
expenditure
financial crises faced by, 66
institutional assistance, 113–114
medical care, 67
non-food consumption
expenditure, 89
nutrition and health care, 67
opting for borrowings, 107
savings and asset holdings, 114
socio-economic categories of,
161–162
total outflow of income, 89
which saved and dissaved at
the same time, 89
human capital, 78
investments, 85
human immunodeficiency virus
(HIV), 2
cases reported/detected in Goa,
5–6
consequences of, 9
detection of, 5
economic impacts of, 171
employment, discrimination
and employer-support, 33
epidemic in India, 3, 183
hospitalization details of, 138

households pertaining to loss of
income, 53
pattern of spread of, 8
prevalence rate, 3
risk of, 176
sexual mode of transmission, 6
transmission rate of, 176
'treatment' aspect of, 177
vaccine for, 174
human rights, 179–180
Human Rights Law Network
(HRLN), 1, 3, 183
human T lymphotropic virus-III
(HTLV-III), 2

iatrogenic poverty, 155, 159
income of HIV+ respondents
compensation, financial, 27
coping mechanisms pertaining
to, 45–47
in female-headed households,
46
impact due to absenteeism
caused by illness, 34–36
impact of HIV/AIDS on, 13–14
loss during the last one year,
48–51
loss on account of death, 42
nature of change in earnings, 31
pertaining to the caregiver,
37–42
from present employment,
32–37
from previous and present
employment, 24–32
primary reasons for changes
in, 30
unrequited and/or unrevealed
income (UUI), 55
institutional assistance, for HIV/
AIDS households, 113–114
Integrated Counselling and
Testing Centres (ICTCs), 5, 174,
201, 204

interest earnings, 17, 56n6
International Committee for
    Nomenclature of Viruses, 2
International Labour Organization
    (ILO), 32, 40

Karnataka, 6, 182
Karnataka Network for Positive
    People (KNP+), 182
Kendall's tau rank correlation,
    203
Kenya, 28, 34
Khan, F., 155

labour productivity, 9, 120, 159
Lawyers Collective, 183
Lazarus Effect, 145
life-expectancy, 159
life insurance policy, 113
lifestyle disease, 175
loans. *See* bank loans
lymphadenopathy associated
    virus (LAV), 2

Maharashtra, 3, 6, 32
male-headed HHs, 45, 63, 98,
    113–114, 204
    annual non-wage income, 18
malnutrition, 67, 174
Mann-Whitney U test, 203
marginalized HHs, 8, 56
medical care, 67, 145, 160, 163
medical discrimination, 163,
    177–178
medical health, medicalization of,
    179
medical insurance, 113–114
'medico-curative' measures, for
    HIV/AIDS infection, 176–179
Millennium Development Goals
    (MDG), 11
moderate prevalence states, 6
Montagnier, Luc, 2
morbidity, 11, 22, 55

mortality, due to HIV/AIDS
    infection, 6, 11, 22, 55, 177
Mother to Child Transmission
    (MTCT), 176, 183

National AIDS Control
    Organization (NACO), 4, 6,
    9–10, 29, 47, 121, 148, 162
National AIDS Control
    Programme (NACP), 183
National Council of Applied
    Economic Research (NCAER),
    9, 29, 121
National Family Health Survey
    (NFHS), 176
National Health Bill (2009), 177
national income (NI), 120
National Rural Employment
    Guarantee Act (NREGA), 181
Nemapare, Prisca, 67
Nigeria, 4, 120
non-governmental organizations
    (NGOs), 11, 29, 34, 61, 65–67, 75,
    78–79, 84, 92, 103, 109, 112, 121,
    130, 151, 172, 202
non-HIV earning members, death
    of
    additional burden on, 42–45
    amount of money spent on
        funerals, 44
    and caregiving duties, 46
    details of, 43
    distribution based on monthly
        income slabs, 44
    in female-headed households, 46
non-hospitalized illness episodes
    (NHIEs), 126–136
    economic impact, 136
    treatment of those frequently/
        continuously ill with, 133
non-hospitalized illness treatment
    (NHIT), 122, 126–136
    duration of, 133
    expenses for, 134

households in terms of total
expenses on, 135
and number of years since
detection of HIV, 130
of those frequently or
continuously sick in the last
month, 132
non-wage income, 17–18, 56n6, 60,
91–92, 94
nutrition
nutritional management, 160
nutritional support, 66

opportunistic infections (OIs), 1–2,
6, 67, 131, 145, 159
availability of drugs for, 177
free medication for, 178
treatment of, 149, 155
orphans, 7, 67, 78, 159, 183
other annual HH consumption
expenditure, 60, 76, 77, 79–80,
82–84, 89, 122–123, 158
out-of-pocket (OOP) expenses, 91,
121, 128, 146–147, 149, 151–152,
154–155

paid work, 115
'partly sponsored' food, 61–62, 66
patients rights, 178
pension/pensioners, 14, 18, 23,
92, 181
people living with HIV/AIDS
(PLWHA), 3–7, 9, 11, 54, 60, 91,
121, 155, 160, 163, 178–180
discrimination against, 178
at workplace, 182
economic conditions of, 181, 183
Focus Group Discussion (FGD),
203
free legal services, 183
guidelines for dispensing health
services to, 179
hurdles faced by, 181
insurance cover to, 182

life expectancy of, 149
medical discrimination faced
by, 163, 168n36
nutritional intervention, 67
pension to, 181
travelling ordeals for, 177
treatment of, 176, 179
perinatal transmission, 8, 176
Population Services International
(PSI), 182
poverty, issue of, 155, 159
below poverty line (BPL), 178,
181–182
and health care, 176
poverty line, 82, 146, 181
prevalence of HIV/AIDS
high, 4, 6
low, 4
moderate, 6
preventive measures, for HIV/
AIDS, 173–176
Price Distribution System (PDS), 66
pricing of drugs, 161
Primary Health Centres (PHC), 130
private treatment, for HIV
infection, 133, 201
prostitution, 8, 103. *See also*
commercial sex workers (CSWs)
Provident Fund (PF), 23
public health systems, 120–121, 178

ration-cards, 66
Red Crescent, 2
Red Cross, 2
registration of marriage, 3, 176,
184n14
regular monthly HH consumption
expenditure, 60, 68–69, 72–73,
75, 76, 84
regular monthly medical treatment
(RMMT), 122, 145–155
ART treatment, 145–149
other RMMT expenses
(excluding ART), 149–151

total RMMT expenses, 152–155
remittances, 84–85
   comparative amount of, 85
rent, 71–72, 201
Report of the National
   Commission on
   Macroeconomics and Health
   (2005), 174
'reverse demographic gift', 22
'Right to Food', 181
right to life, 183
rural health centres, equipment and
   employee absenteeism in, 177

school education, 78, 91
Schoub, Barry D., 174
second-line treatment, 161, 167n31,
   177
self employment, 115, 210
sex education, 175
sexually transmitted disease/
   infection (STD/STI), 8
sexual mode of HIV transmission,
   6–8
short message service (SMS), 179
social justice, 179–180
social security system, 11, 27, 55,
   113
socio-economic impact of HIV/
   AIDS, 9, 19, 94
South Africa, 3–4, 19, 22, 54, 60, 91,
   185n15
Spearman's rank correlation, 203
spending, on treatment and care, 11
Star Health, 182
Sub-Saharan Africa, 2–3, 120
suicide, 66
supply of drugs, 177

Tamil Nadu, 175
third-line treatment, 161, 167n31
time poverty, 42
total annual HH consumption
   expenditure, 122, 158–159

total annual HH income, 18, 24,
   47, 51, 54, 63–64, 73, 84–85, 88,
   91–94, 107, 111, 157–158, 170–171
tourism, 10
transmission of AIDS/HIVs, 6–8
travelling expenditure, overview
   of, 73–75
tuberculosis (TB), 167n33, 185n17

un-affordability, 47, 55, 78
unemployment, 29, 45, 49, 51
United Nations Development
   Programme (UNDP), 1, 29, 121,
   180
United Nations Millennium
   Summit (2000), 11
United Progressive Alliance-II
   (UPA-II), 181
unorganized sector, 27, 172
unrequited and/or unrevealed
   income (UUI), 55, 64, 79, 88,
   103–104, 107, 170–171
   comparative profile of, 104
unskilled labour, 10–11, 29, 34
unskilled labour sector, AIDS
   epidemic in, 10

vaccine, for HIV/AIDS, 174–175
Vatra Bhet scheme, 182
viral load, 75, 145–147, 162

wage earners, HIV/AIDS impact
   on, 31–32
wage income, 17, 41, 51
widows, 18, 92, 115, 181
women's education, return on
   investment in, 174
Work Force Participation Rate
   (WFPR), 46–47
World Bank, 2, 138, 173, 175
World Health Organisation
   (WHO), 2–4, 7, 175, 179
   'treat 3 million by 2005' ('3 by 5')
   programme, 179

About the Author

Savio P. Falleiro is Associate Professor and senior faculty member at Rosary College of Commerce and Arts, Navelim (Goa), India. Dr Falleiro is also the Vice Principal and Head of the Department of Economics at the same college. He has 24 years of teaching experience. He was awarded the degree of Doctor of Philosophy in Economics by Goa University (India) for his work related to the study of the economic implications of HIV/AIDS on individuals and households. He has been an avid writer and has published numerous research-based articles.

In 2008–2009, he was granted a Minor Research Project by the University Grants Commission for his study related to HIV/AIDS awareness among college students. Over the years he has contributed in various capacities to the academic arena, including being a resource person, guest faculty at the MBA programme and member of different academic and non-academic bodies.